D0271345

# Design and Analysis of Cluster Randomization Trials in Health Research

First published in Great Britain in 2000 by
Arnold, a member of the Hodder Headline Group,
338 Euston Road, London NW1 3BH

**http://www.arnoldpublishers.com**

Co-published in the United States of America by
Oxford University Press Inc.,
198 Madison Avenue, New York, NY 10016



*British Library Cataloguing in Publication Data*
A catalogue record for this book is available from the British Library

*Library of Congress Cataloging-in-Publication Data*
A catalog record for this book is available from the Library of Congress

ISBN: 0 340 69153 0

1 2 3 4 5 6 7 8 9 10

Commissioning Editor: Liz Gooster
Production Editor: Anke Ueberberg
Production Controller: Fiona Byrne
Cover Design: Terry Griffiths

Typeset in 10/12 pt Times by Academic + Technical, Bristol
Printed and bound by Redwood Books, Trowbridge

# Design and Analysis of Cluster Randomization Trials in Health Research


**Allan Donner**
**Professor and Chair**
**Department of Epidemiology and Biostatistics**
**The University of Western Ontario, Canada**

**Neil Klar**
**Senior Biostatistician**
**Division of Preventive Oncology**
**Cancer Care Ontario**
**Toronto, Ontario, Canada**


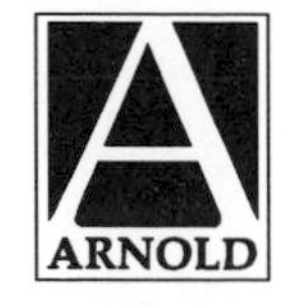



A member of the Hodder Headline Group
LONDON

This book is dedicated to the memory of Dr Martin Bass, a superb scientist and beloved friend and colleague.

# Contents

# Acknowledgements

We each have many thanks to offer. Allan Donner's work on this book began over the 1997–1998 academic year during a one-year study leave generously granted by the University of Western Ontario. He also received funding support from the Natural Sciences and Engineering Research Council of Canada that was much appreciated. From 1997 to 1999, Neil Klar received support from a faculty grant provided by the Schering-Plough Corporation and the Department of Biostatistics at the Harvard School of Public Health.

The book could not have been completed without the assistance of several important people. Dr Mekibib Altaye of the University of Western Ontario, Dr Gilda Piaggio of the Special Programme of Research, Development and Research Training in Human Reproduction at the World Health Organization, and Dr Walter Hauck of Thomas Jefferson University provided a careful reading that substantially improved the book. Dr Stan Shapiro of McGill University, Dr Pei Liu of Xuzhou Medical College and Dr Guangyong Zou of the University of Western Ontario also provided helpful comments. Invaluable secretarial assistance was provided by Ms Clara Fernandes and Ms Donna Shiplett, with dedicated administrative support supplied by Mrs Gloria Murphy. The enduring patience and unflagging encouragement of our editors, Ms Nikki Dennis and Ms Kirsty Stroud, has also been much appreciated.

Particular thanks are owed to Dr David Murray of the University of Memphis for providing access to his study data on adolescent tobacco use.

We also want to thank our families without whose love and support this book would not exist. In particular, Allan Donner would like to thank his wife Brenda and daughter Katharine, and Neil Klar would like to thank his parents, Irma and Gus.

# Preface

A cluster randomization trial is one in which intact social units, or clusters of individuals, rather than individuals themselves, are randomized to different intervention groups. Trials randomizing clusters, sometimes called group randomization trials, have become particularly widespread in the evaluation of non-therapeutic interventions, including lifestyle modification, educational programmes and innovations in the provision of health care. The units of randomization in such studies are diverse, ranging from relatively small clusters, such as households or families, to entire neighbourhoods or communities, but also including worksites, hospital wards, classrooms and medical practices. There are also reports of trials that have randomized more unusual units, including athletic teams (Walsh *et al.* 1999), tribes (Glasgow *et al.* 1995a), religious institutions (Lasater *et al.* 1997) and sex establishments (Fontanet *et al.* 1998).

The increasing popularity of this design among health researchers over the past two decades has led to an extensive body of methodology and a growing, although somewhat scattered, literature that cuts across several disciplines in the statistical, social and medical sciences. The purpose of this book is to present a systematic and unified treatment of this topic, so that it may be used as a reference source for investigators in the planning or analysis stages of a study. It also may be used as a textbook for a graduate level course in research methodology aimed at biostatisticians, epidemiologists, health service researchers and public health professionals. The overall prerequisite for the book is an understanding of the fundamentals of biostatistics at the level of Armitage and Berry (1994) or Rosner (1995). Familiarity with the basic principles of design and analysis of clinical trials, as may be found, for example, in standard texts such as Friedman *et al.* (1996) or Pocock (1983), is also assumed.

Given the ready availability of several excellent textbooks on clinical trial design and analysis, the question may well be raised as to whether a separate text on cluster randomized trials is required. We would argue that it is, given that well-established methods for the design and analysis of clinical trials are incomplete, and in some cases potentially misleading, if applied to trials randomizing intact social units. The clustering of subjects within these units implies that standard approaches to sample size estimation, statistical analysis and the reporting of trial results cannot be directly applied.

The first four chapters are fairly non-technical and begin with a general introduction to cluster randomization trials (Ch. 1). The historical development of these trials is discussed in Chapter 2. Issues relevant to the planning of cluster randomization trials and to their ethical challenges are dealt with in Chapters 3 and 4, respectively.

The chapters dealing with sample size estimation (Ch. 5) and data analysis (Chs 6–8) are more quantitatively oriented, although we have attempted to make them as accessible as possible to readers who are familiar with basic statistical concepts and methods. Numerous worked examples have been included to clarify their application to cluster randomization trials. Methods for the analysis of binary outcome data are presented in Chapter 6, while Chapter 7 deals with methods for the analysis of quantitative outcomes. Relatively new developments in the field of cluster randomization, such as the analysis of time-to-event and count data, are described in Chapter 8. The order and detail of each chapter reflect the relative frequency with which these different types of outcome data are encountered in cluster randomization trials.

The final chapter (Ch. 9) of the text returns to less technical material, presenting guidelines for trial reporting. This chapter also provides a summary of many of the key issues raised in previous chapters.

Each week brings new methodological developments in the field of cluster randomization. As a consequence, a challenge we faced in writing this book was in deciding at what point we should stop. For example, the growing number of trials adopting this design has led to an increased interest in conducting meta-analyses that synthesize the results of trials that may involve different units of random assignment (e.g. Fawzi *et al.* 1993, Rooney and Murray 1996). Economic evaluation of cluster randomization trials should also receive more attention in the future. While inclusion of such largely undeveloped topics is beyond the scope of the present text, we fully expect important progress on these topics in the near future.

Software for many of the sample size and analysis formulas presented in this book has been prepared by Mr Alain Pinol and Dr Gilda Piaggio of the UNDP/UNFPA/WHO World Bank Special Programme of Research, Development and Training in Human Reproduction at the World Health Organization, Geneva, Switzerland. Details on obtaining this software, much of which is not available in standard statistical packages, can be obtained from the Arnold Publishing web page: http://www.arnoldpublishers.com/support/cluster.

Pocock (1996) has stated 'with increasing use of cluster randomization, especially in developing country intervention trials, there is a need for their methodological foundation to be more thoroughly understood'. This book is an attempt to provide such a foundation.

# 1

# Introduction

In this introductory chapter we deal with the basic issues that must be addressed when investigators first consider adopting a cluster randomization design. Foremost among these is the justification for adopting cluster randomization, given its lack of efficiency and weaker statistical power relative to a design individually randomizing the same number of subjects. This topic is discussed in Section 1.1. A second issue, considered in Sections 1.2 and 1.3, is the inevitable impact of cluster randomization on the methodology of the trial, ranging from sample size estimation to analysis, but also encompassing standard design issues such as the role of stratification or matching.

The last three sections of this chapter are intended to place the overall discussion in context. Section 1.4 indicates why we have decided to focus specifically on randomized trials, while Section 1.5 introduces the effect of the unit of inference on study design and data analysis. Section 1.6 explains our preference for using the term 'cluster randomization' rather than other terms that have sometimes been used to refer to this design.

## 1.1 Why randomize clusters?

The statistical features of cluster randomization were first brought to wide attention in the health research community by Cornfield (1978). His paper made it clear that such allocation schemes are less efficient, in a statistical sense, than designs which randomize individuals to intervention groups. However, this general result was recognized much earlier in the statistical literature (see Walsh 1947). The loss of efficiency arises because the responses of individuals in an intact cluster tend to be more similar than the responses of individuals in different clusters. This is perhaps why, as pointed out by McKinlay *et al.* (1989), the theory of experimental design as developed by Sir Ronald Fisher (1935) assumes, without exception, that the experimental unit which is randomized is also the unit of analysis. This is not necessarily the case in a cluster randomization trial, which is one of its principal distinguishing characteristics.

The degree of similarity among responses within a cluster is typically measured by a parameter known as the intracluster (intraclass) correlation coefficient. Denoted by the Greek letter $\rho$, this parameter may be interpreted as the standard Pearson correlation coefficient between any two responses in the same cluster. As shown in Section 1.3, stating that $\rho$ is positive is equivalent to assuming that the variation between observations in different clusters exceeds the variation within clusters. Under these conditions, we may say that the design is characterized by 'between-cluster variation'. Using terminology suggested by Whiting-O'Keefe *et al.* (1984), this is also equivalent to stating that clusters cannot be assumed to be 'interchangeable' with regard to the experimental endpoint. The underlying reasons for lack of interchangeability or variation between clusters will differ from trial to trial, but in practice may include the following:

- *Subject selection, where individuals are in a position to choose the cluster to which they belong*. For example, in a trial randomizing medical practices, the characteristics of patients belonging to a practice could be related to age or sex differences among physicians. To the extent that these characteristics are also related to patient response, a clustering effect will be induced within practices. In addition, as noted by Rhee *et al.* (1980), the outcomes on two or more patients treated by the same physician could share the influence of that physician's style of practice. Similar selection factors may operate in worksite trials, where employees and employers may choose each other on the basis of specific characteristics, such as socioeconomic status or ethnic affiliation (Kelder *et al.* 1993). In trials randomizing large communities or counties, geographical selection factors may also play a role, e.g. when older people seek to reside in warmer climates, or when patients with respiratory problems migrate to less humid regions of the country. As Koepsell (1998) pointed out, 'individuals often choose to reside in a given community because they have characteristics in common with other community residents and thus "fit in". Those characteristics may, in turn, be associated with the health behaviours of interest'.
- *The influence of covariates at the cluster level, where all individuals in a cluster are affected in a similar manner as a result of sharing exposure to a common environment*. For example, it is known that postoperative medical outcomes, including complications and mortality, may vary systematically among surgeons (McArdle and Hole 1991). More generally, as pointed out by Divine *et al.* (1992), there 'may be considerable variation in patient care behaviour from provider to provider due to differences in attitude or in amounts of knowledge absorbed'. Bland and Kerry (1997) note that the effect of clustering may be particularly strong in health care trials in which the intervention is applied to the provider of care rather than to the patient directly. This is because the between-cluster variation will then reflect variation in the responses of individual practitioners, as well as variation due to differences among patients. As an example, they cite the trial reported by White *et al.* (1987), which was designed to improve the treatment of asthma in general practice through a programme of physician education.

  The structural features of an environment may also induce a clustering effect. For example, infection rates in nurseries may vary owing to differences in temperature or other environmental conditions, while differences in by-laws between municipalities could influence the success of smoking cessation programmes. As pointed out by Rice and Leyland (1996), patients attending the same hospital may share several common influences, e.g. the same pressure to shorten length of stay. Finally, when intact families or households are randomized, the combined effect of both environmental and genetic factors will contribute to the observed between-cluster variation.

- *The tendency of infectious diseases to spread more rapidly within families than between families or throughout communities.* The possibility of outbreaks or epidemics in some clusters, the method by which the infectious agent is spread and its virulence will also affect the degree of between-cluster variation in rates of disease (Smith and Morrow 1991, pp. 24–25).
- *The effect of personal interactions among cluster members who receive the same intervention.* For example, educational strategies or therapies provided in a group setting could lead to a sharing of information or predispositions that create a clustering effect. More generally, as noted by Koepsell (1998), just as infectious agents can be spread from person to person, the transmission of attitudes, norms and behaviours among people who are in regular contact can result in similar responses.

Without extensive empirical data, it is usually impossible to distinguish among the potential reasons for between-cluster variation. Regardless of the specific cause, however, such variation invariably leads to a reduction in the effective sample size for the trial, where the size of the reduction increases with both the magnitude of $\rho$ and the average cluster size. This in turn leads to a loss of precision in estimating the effect of intervention.

Given this loss of efficiency relative to individual randomization, the reasons for adopting a cluster randomization design must clearly rest on other considerations, usually related to ethical issues, the desire to control costs or attempts to minimize experimental contamination. Judging from the published literature, a variety of feasibility considerations and/or the need to minimize or remove contamination appear to be particularly common concerns. For example, Sommer *et al.* (1986) report on a study evaluating the effect of vitamin A supplementation on childhood mortality. In this trial, 450 villages in Indonesia were randomly assigned either to participate in vitamin A supplementation or to serve as a control. Cluster randomization was adopted because it was 'not considered politically feasible' to randomize individuals. It may also be noted that randomization of intact villages avoided the contamination that could have arisen if individuals within a village randomly assigned to different interventions were to share the same medication.

Worksite and hospital-based trials have cited similar concerns. For example, in a multifactorial trial for the prevention of coronary heart disease (Rose 1970, World Health Organization European Collaborative Group 1986), factories were chosen as the unit of randomization to minimize the likelihood of subjects in different intervention groups sharing information concerning preventive advice on coronary risk factors. Similar considerations arose in the design of a trial to determine whether suckling immediately after birth reduces the frequency of postpartum haemorrhage (Bullough *et al.* 1989). Randomization into early suckling and control groups was by birth attendant rather than patient in order 'to reduce the likelihood of contamination of the treatment groups by knowledge of the intervention reaching women awaiting delivery'. This form of contamination is particularly likely to occur when the same personnel are asked to administer both the experimental and control interventions to different patients. An additional concern regarding the feasibility of individual randomization was that the birth attendant 'might not have followed the randomization procedure through misunderstanding its significance'.

The trade-off between the lower precision associated with cluster randomization and the potential contamination bias associated with individual randomization is a factor that frequently arises in the decision to adopt a cluster randomization design. In some trials, the net effect of this trade-off can be estimated quantitatively, e.g. when the contamination is expected only to dilute or attenuate the effect of intervention. Although several mechanisms might well account for such dilution, a particularly simple model that may help in the choice of design is to assume that a certain proportion of control group subjects will, through an extreme form of contamination, 'behave' like experimental group subjects. In this case, guidelines for determining the magnitude of the trade-off between bias and precision have been given by Slymen and Hovell (1997). The resulting decision to adopt cluster or individual randomization is shown to depend on the sizes of the clusters randomized, the value of $\rho$ and the expected degree of contamination.

Of course, the selection of a cluster randomization design does not guarantee that the threat of contamination will be entirely removed. This threat can sometimes be further minimized, however, by implementing the study in a geographic area in which only distinct and well separated clusters of subjects are recruited. This strategy was adopted by Grosskurth *et al.* (1995), who evaluated the impact of improved services for the treatment of sexually transmitted diseases on the incidence of HIV infection in a region of Tanzania, Africa. For this trial, the investigators selected only clusters that comprised relatively large units, each consisting of a population served by a single health centre and its satellites, thereby reducing the contamination that could occur if closely adjacent units were allocated to the experimental and control groups. A similar strategy was employed in the design of the COMMIT trial (Gail *et al.* 1992), where 'the paired communities were geographically close enough to permit monitoring and intervention by the investigators, but not so close that educational activities in the intervention community would affect the control community'.

An additional strategy that has occasionally been used to assess the effect of contamination is to incorporate control group clusters into the design that are external to the experimental trial. This approach was adopted by Schlegel (1977), who evaluated educational programmes for the prevention of adolescent alcohol use and abuse. Classrooms within each of two schools were randomly assigned to various intervention groups. Because of a concern that there could be 'treatment spillage', the overall design also included two control classes from another non-participating school.

Basic feasibility considerations were cited by Bass *et al.* (1986) in their choice of a cluster randomized design for evaluating a programme to enhance the effectiveness of hypertension screening and management in general practice. It was recognized that such a programme would not function effectively if some patients in a practice but not others were entered into it. Therefore in this study the unit of randomization was the physician's practice, with 17 practices assigned to each of the two intervention groups. Similar concerns led to the assignment of clusters of women scheduled to receive maternity care from an obstetrician, clinic or hospital during recruitment (Grant *et al.* 1989).

Randomization of intact practices in these studies, aside from simplifying the trial organization, also avoids that form of contamination which may arise when knowledge of the experimental intervention on the part of the physician and/or other staff either inadvertently or deliberately influences subjects in the control group. The risks associated with individual randomization will be particularly great when the intervention is unblinded, since patients receiving the control intervention may feel disadvantaged as compared with patients who are treated by the same physician but receive a new form of care.

These issues arose in the Edinburgh trial of breast cancer, where the investigators chose to randomize intact general practices rather than individual patients to an experimental or control group (Alexander *et al.* 1989). Aside from the practical problem that there was no adequate list of patients to use as a sampling frame within practices, there was also a concern that contamination of the two arms could arise if control women became aware of fellow patients having been screened and, as a consequence, insisted on screening for themselves. A particularly compelling reason, however, was the investigators' belief that individual randomization would not be acceptable to general practitioners and their patients. This point was made even more strongly by Paci and Alexander (1997), who stated that:

> women invited to screening will wish to discuss with their general practitioner (GP) whether or not to accept; if only half of a particular GP's patients have been (randomly) invited, this may cause practical problems to the GP and lead to resentment on the part of the women who were not invited.

Other practical considerations may also dictate the choice of this design. For example, Farr *et al.* (1988) randomized intact families in an intervention trial designed to evaluate the effectiveness of treated nasal tissues versus placebo tissues in reducing the incidence of respiratory illness. Families rather than individuals were allocated in this trial in order to enhance compliance, which was thought to be more likely if all members of a family were assigned the same treatment regimen.

More generally, cluster randomization may be attractive in trials of infectious diseases where the aim of the study is to reduce transmission of infection. Individual randomization might prove impractical because the dynamics of transmission might lead some subjects not receiving the intervention nevertheless to receive protection as a consequence of herd immunity (Comstock 1978, Smith and Morrow 1991, Hayes 1998). The risk would be even greater in trials of live attenuated vaccines (e.g. Pollock 1966).

In each of the above examples, the investigators chose to adopt a cluster randomization design in order to avoid ethical, logistical or methodological problems that might otherwise have arisen. In some studies, however, randomization by cluster is the only natural choice or a clear necessity, with no special justification required. Thus, as stated by Dunn (1994), 'it is often impossible to introduce an innovative service or change in administration to only part of a service and leave the rest as it is'. This was arguably the case in the HIV prevention trial described above (Grosskurth *et al.* 1995). As the authors note, randomization was necessary at the community level since the intervention involved the provision of improved services at designated health facilities, with these services available to the entire population served by each facility. The CATCH study (Zucker *et al.* 1995), a large-scale community health trial for the prevention of cardiovascular disease, is another example. These investigators chose to randomize schools to intervention groups because 'CATCH interventions are designed to be implemented on a school wide basis, en bloc to students in a given school'.

Intervention programmes that use mass education are similarly circumscribed, since one cannot generally provide general exhortations concerning diet, smoking or exercise to some people and not to others in the same community. This was the case in the COMMIT trial (COMMIT Research Group 1995a, b), designed to study an intervention to accelerate smoking cessation among heavy smokers and to reduce smoking prevalence. Health care providers and employers were encouraged to promote smoking cessation, as accompanied by public education and media campaigns. As discussed by Gail *et al.* (1996), these community-based interventions had the potential to affect every smoker in the community, thus precluding individual randomization within communities. As further explained by Byar (1988):

> it is known that heavy smokers experience great difficulty in giving up smoking when the usual methods focused on individuals are used. Cluster randomization was chosen, based upon the hypothesis that heavy smokers will find it easier to stop smoking when cessation assistance is made widely available in an environment where smoking is made less socially acceptable.

Other examples of trials employing cluster randomization when the intervention is naturally applied on a community-wide or geographic basis are given by Smith and Morrow (1991) and Raudenbush (1997).

## 1.2 What is the impact of cluster randomization on the design and analysis of a trial?

As previously noted, Fisher's classical theory of experimental design assumes, without exception, that the experimental unit which is randomized is also the unit of analysis. Many of the challenges of cluster randomization arise because inferences are frequently intended to apply at the individual level, while randomization is at the cluster level. If inferences were intended to apply at the cluster level, implying that an analysis at the cluster level would also be most appropriate, the study could be regarded, at least with respect to adopting an approach to the sample size estimation and analysis, as a standard clinical trial. However, if individual-level analyses are to be performed, the lack of statistical independence among members in a cluster will invalidate standard approaches to both the estimation of sample size and the analysis of the trial data. Application of standard sample size formulas will, in general, lead to underpowered studies, which may, as a consequence, be inconclusive. On the other hand, application of standard methods to the statistical analysis, which invariably assume no between-cluster variation, will tend to bias observed $p$-values downward, thus risking a spurious claim of statistical significance. This problem has led to the famous quote in the epidemiological literature by Cornfield (1978) that 'randomization by cluster accompanied by an analysis appropriate to randomization by individual is an exercise in self-deception and should be discouraged'. Similar points have also been made frequently in the educational literature (e.g. Zucker 1990). However, self-deception of this sort may be psychologically difficult to resist if the investigator believes the resulting analysis will yield an increased ability to detect small intervention effects, especially if it is also believed that the stated objection is merely a methodological nicety. It can only be argued in response that such analyses are invalid, and in fact are a principal reason why many trials reported as statistically significant in the literature may well be non-significant. It may also be added that randomization by cluster accompanied by a sample size assessment appropriate to randomization by individual is also an exercise in self-deception. While the former may lead to a type I error substantially above that which is planned for, the latter may lead to a substantially elevated type II error.

Unfortunately, many cluster randomization trials routinely fail to take into account between-cluster variation in both the design and the analysis. For example, a review of 21 primary prevention trials using cluster randomization reported by Simpson *et al.* (1995) showed that between-cluster variation was accounted for in the sample size or power calculations by only four of the studies (19 per cent), and accounted for in the analysis by only 12 (57 per cent). These results are almost identical to those reported in an earlier review by Donner *et al.* (1990). These authors found that only three of 16 trials reviewed (19 per cent) accounted for between-cluster variation in the sample size planning, while eight trials (50 per cent) took account of the clustering in the analysis. Other methodological reviews of cluster randomization trials (e.g. Butler and Bachmann 1996, Rooney and Murray 1996) have shown similar disappointing results.

Some authors who have failed to account for between-cluster variation in the design and analysis of their trials appear to have recognized the theoretical importance of this issue, while discounting its practical importance for their own study. For example, investigators in a trial which randomized households of children to receive either vitamin A supplementation or placebo (Stansfield *et al.* 1993) chose to ignore the possibility of between-household variation with respect to morbidity on the grounds that a 'negligible design effect was expected'. Unless supported by strong empirical evidence, this would seem a risky assumption to make. We discuss this issue further in Section 1.3.

Although the impact of cluster randomization is perhaps most dramatically felt on sample size considerations and on the required approach to the statistical analysis, several other issues related to the conduct and interpretation of clinical trials are also affected. These include issues related to the role of stratification, subject blindness and informed consent, as well as special problems regarding the tracking of subjects and loss to follow-up. We discuss these issues further in Chapters 3–5.

## 1.3 Quantifying the effect of clustering

Consider an experimental trial in which $k$ clusters of $m$ individuals are randomly assigned to each of an experimental group and a control group. We suppose that the primary aim of the trial is to compare the groups with respect to their mean values on a normally distributed response variable $Y$ having a common but unknown variance $\sigma^2$. Appropriate estimates of the population means $\mu_1$ and $\mu_2$ are given by the usual sample means $\overline{Y}_1$ and $\overline{Y}_2$ for the experimental and control groups, respectively, where these estimates are computed over all individuals in each group. From a well-known result in cluster sampling (e.g. Moser and Kalton 1972), the variance of each of these means is given by

$$\mathrm{Var}(\overline{Y}_i) = \frac{\sigma^2}{km}[1 + (m - 1)\rho], \qquad i = 1, 2 \tag{1.1}$$

where $\rho$ is the intracluster correlation coefficient defined in Section 1.1. At $\rho = 0$, equation (1.1) reduces to the standard expression for the variance of a sample mean that applies under simple random sampling. If $\sigma^2$ is replaced by $P(1 - P)$, where $P$ denotes the probability of a success, equation (1.1) also provides an expression for the variance of a sample proportion under clustering.

For sample size determination, equation (1.1) implies that the usual estimate of the required number of individuals in each group should be multiplied by the variance inflation factor, $IF = 1 + (m - 1)\rho$, to provide the same statistical power as would be obtained by randomizing $km$ individuals to each group when there is no clustering effect. This expression is also well-known in the sample survey literature, in which it is referred to as a 'design effect' (Kish 1965). The special case $\rho = 0$ corresponds to that of statistical independence among members of a cluster. The case $\rho = 1$, on the other hand, corresponds to total dependence. In this case, all responses in a cluster are identical, so that the total information supplied by the cluster is no more than that supplied by a single member, i.e. the 'effective cluster size' is one. In general, the effective cluster size is given by the simple formula $m/[1 + (m - 1)\rho] = m/IF$. In the case of variable cluster sizes, substituting the average cluster size $\overline{m}$ for $m$ in $IF$ will underestimate the variance of $\overline{Y}_i$, but only slightly unless the variation in cluster sizes is large.

As stated in Section 1.1, the parameter $\rho$ may be interpreted as the usual pairwise correlation coefficient between any two members of the same cluster. If we add the additional assumption that the intracluster correlation cannot be negative, $\rho$ may also be interpreted as the proportion of overall variation in response that can be accounted for by the between-cluster variation. With this interpretation, we may write $\rho = \sigma_A^2/\sigma^2 = \sigma_A^2/(\sigma_A^2 + \sigma_W^2)$, where $\sigma_A^2$ is the between-cluster component of variance and $\sigma_W^2$ the within-cluster component. The variance of a group mean can then be written as $\mathrm{Var}(\overline{Y}_i) = (\sigma_A^2 + \sigma_W^2/m)/k$. Note also we may write $\sigma_W^2 = \sigma^2(1 - \rho)$, indicating that the effect of a positive intracluster correlation coefficient is to reduce the within-cluster variance by a factor $1 - \rho$. This reduction in variance is what creates the enhanced similarity in response among members of the same cluster.

Of course, the clusters recruited to participate in a trial, as well as the individuals sampled within clusters, will rarely be selected in a truly random fashion from a well-defined population. Therefore this population is usually conceptualized as hypothetical, with judgment playing an important role when interpreting the values of both $\rho$ and the variance components $\sigma_A^2$ and $\sigma_W^2$.

A sample estimate of $\rho$ may be obtained by performing a standard one-way analysis of variance among and within clusters (e.g. Snedecor and Cochran 1989, Section

13.5). Consider the case of a single sample of $k$ clusters, each of size $m$, and denote the mean square error among and within clusters by MSC and MSW respectively. Then the 'analysis of variance' estimator of $\rho$ is given by

$$\hat{\rho} = \frac{\text{MSC} - \text{MSW}}{\text{MSC} + (m-1)\text{MSW}} = S_{\text{A}}^2/(S_{\text{A}}^2 + S_{\text{W}}^2) \tag{1.2}$$

where and $S_{\text{A}}^2 = (\text{MSC} - \text{MSW})/m$ and $S_{\text{W}}^2 = \text{MSW}$ are sample estimates of $\sigma_{\text{A}}^2$ and $\sigma_{\text{W}}^2$ respectively.

For the case of variable cluster sizes $m_j$, $j = 1, 2, \ldots, k$, $m$ may be replaced by

$$m_0 = \left(\frac{1}{k-1}\right)\left(M - \sum_{j=1}^{k} m_j^2/M\right)$$

where $M = \sum_{j=1}^{k} m_j$ denotes the total number of individuals in the sample. Rewriting $m_0$ as

$$\overline{m} - \sum_{j=1}^{k} \frac{(m_j - \overline{m})^2}{(k-1)M}$$

shows that $m_0$ is always slightly less than the average cluster size $\bar{m} = M/k$ although only slightly less if $k$ is large.

For clusters of the same size $m$, $\hat{\rho}$ is virtually identical to the 'pairwise' estimator of $\rho$ obtained by computing the usual Pearson product–moment correlation over all possible pairs of observations that can be created within clusters. Otherwise, $\hat{\rho}$ can be shown to be the more accurate estimator of $\rho$, particularly when the cluster sizes are highly variable (Donner and Koval 1980).

Equation (1.2) also applies to the case of a binary response variable, with the observation $Y$ denoted, say, by 1 (success) or 0 (failure). The estimator of $\rho$ may then be written, for reasonably large $k$, as

$$\hat{\rho} = 1 - \frac{\sum_{j=1}^{k} m_j \hat{P}_j (1 - \hat{P}_j)}{k(\overline{m} - 1)\hat{P}(1 - \hat{P})}$$

where $\hat{P}_j$ denotes the proportion of successes in the $j$th cluster, $j = 1, 2, \ldots, k$, and

$$\hat{P} = \frac{\sum_{j=1}^{k} m_j \hat{P}_j}{\sum_{j=1}^{k} m_j}$$

is the overall proportion of successes. It is also interesting to note that $\hat{\rho}$ is a version of the kappa statistic commonly used to estimate the degree of interobserver agreement among a set of raters with respect to a binary trait measured repeatedly on each of $k$ subjects ($m_j$ raters observing the $j$th subject, $j = 1, 2, \ldots, k$). This identity shows the close relationship between measures of interobserver agreement, where the similarity among ratings taken on the same subject is of prime interest, and more general measures of intracluster correlation. Detailed discussion of $\hat{\rho}$ in the context of measuring interobserver agreement is given by Fleiss (1981, Section 13.2).

Since negative values of $\rho$ are considered to be implausible in most cluster randomization trials, it is common practice to set $\hat{\rho} = 0$ if $\hat{\rho}$ is computed as negative in any given sample. Such truncation is equivalent to assuming that the observed negative value may be attributed to chance (although see remark 2. at the end of this section).

In most applications, values of $\rho$ are small and positive. However, it must be emphasized that the effect of clustering depends on the joint influence of both $m$ and $\rho$. Failure to appreciate this point has led to the occasional suggestion in the epidemiological and clinical literature that clustering may be detected or ruled out on the basis of testing the value of $\hat{\rho}$ for statistical significance, i.e. testing $H_0: \rho = 0$ versus $H_1: \rho > 0$ (e.g. Cambien *et al.* 1981, Kramer 1988, p. 84). The weakness of this approach is that values of $\hat{\rho}$ may be very small in practice, particularly for the large clusters which are typically recruited in community intervention trials. Therefore the power of a test for detecting such values as statistically significant tends to be unacceptably low in practice (e.g. Donner and Klar 1996). Yet small values of $\rho$, combined with large cluster sizes, can yield sizeable design effects, which, if unaccounted for, can seriously disturb the validity of standard statistical procedures. Thus we would recommend that investigators inherently assume the existence of intracluster correlation, a well-documented phenomenon, rather than attempt to rule it out using statistical testing procedures. This advice is also consistent with the well-accepted strategy of adopting an analytic approach that corresponds to the study design.

Extensive reviews of proposed estimators of intracluster correlation are given by Donner (1986) for continuous data and by Ridout *et al.* (1999) for binary data.

## Further remarks

1. The definition of $\rho$ in terms of proportion of variation explained is easily extended to studies in which clustering is expected to arise at more than one level. For example, in school-based studies (e.g. Siddiqui *et al.* 1996), two intracluster correlations are frequently defined, reflecting (a) the variation among schools, and (b) the variation among classrooms within schools. Let the total variance be denoted by $\sigma^2 = \sigma_S^2 + \sigma_C^2 + \sigma_W^2$, where $\sigma_S^2$ is the between-school component of variance, $\sigma_C^2$ is the variance component among classrooms within schools, and $\sigma_W^2$ is the within-classroom component of variance. Then the intracluster correlation for students within schools (between classrooms) is defined as

$$\rho_S = \frac{\sigma_S^2}{\sigma_S^2 + \sigma_C^2 + \sigma_W^2}$$

while the intracluster correlation for students within classrooms is defined as

$$\rho_C = \frac{\sigma_S^2 + \sigma_C^2}{\sigma_S^2 + \sigma_C^2 + \sigma_W^2}$$

These definitions imply $\rho_C \geqslant \rho_S$, reflecting the greater similarity to be expected among students in the same classroom than among students merely in the same school.

2. The interpretation of $\rho$ in terms of proportion of variation explained also assumes, by definition, that $\rho \geqslant 0$. However, the interpretation of $\rho$ as the pairwise correlation coefficient between any two members of the same cluster is slightly more general in that it permits negative values of $\rho$ to be interpreted. (For non-negative values of $\rho$, the two interpretations are essentially equivalent.) Although values of $\rho$ less than zero in cluster randomization studies are rare, they are theoretically possible. Kelder *et al.* (1993) give an interpretation of a negative intracluster correlation coefficient in the context of a worksite intervention trial in which persons within a worksite are less similar to one another than they are to persons in another worksite. This can occur, for example, if competition between members within a worksite leads to an increase in heterogeneity with respect to the outcome variable of interest. Competitive mechanisms among cluster members may also be observed to generate negative intracluster correlations in teratological studies that randomize intact litters of laboratory animals to different treatment groups (Marubini *et al.* 1988).
3. We have described above the impact of cluster randomization on the variance of sample means and proportions. The corresponding impact on other frequently calculated simple statistics may also be quantified. For example, consider the simple regression of a dependent variable $Y$, either continuous or binary, on a single individual-level covariate $X$, where all clusters are of the same size $m$. Scott and Holt (1982), for the case of a continuous dependent variable, and Neuhaus and Segal (1993), for the case of a dichotomous outcome variable, showed that the variance of the estimated regression coefficient of $Y$ on $X$ is inflated as a consequence of the clustering effect by the factor $IF_R = 1 + (m-1)\rho_X \rho$, where $\rho$ is the intracluster correlation coefficient with respect to the outcome variable $Y$, and $\rho_X$ is the intracluster correlation coefficient with respect to the covariate $X$. Note that if $X$ is a cluster-level covariate (e.g. representing intervention group) then $\rho_X = 1$ and $IF_R$ reduces to the more familiar expression $IF$. For individual level covariates, however, $IF_R < IF$, showing that the effect of clustering on the variances of estimated regression coefficients is generally less severe than on the variances of estimated means and proportions. Nonetheless, it is obvious that if $m$ is sizeable, the clustering effect may still be substantial in practice.

## 1.4 Randomized versus non-randomized comparisons

The advantages of random allocation in cluster randomization trials are the same as in clinical trials randomizing individuals. These include the assurance that selection bias has played no role in the assignment of clusters to different interventions, the balancing, in an average sense, of baseline characteristics in the different intervention groups, and the formal justification for the application of statistical distribution theory to the analysis of results. Thus randomized trials are generally regarded as the 'gold standard' for the evaluation of intervention. Nonetheless, there has been considerable discussion, particularly in the area of community intervention trials, as to the relative merits of randomized versus non-randomized allocation schemes. The reasons given for non-randomized allocation, or 'quasi-experimentation' as it is sometimes referred to, are usually very practical in nature, as related to political considerations, feasibility and cost. These reasons are, of course, very similar to those cited for the allocation of clusters rather than individuals at an earlier decision point. There may even be perceived methodological advantages to non-randomized trials. For example, the systematic allocation of geographically separated control and intervention clusters might be seen as necessary to alleviate concerns regarding experimental contamination. There may also be occasions when the benefits of intervention are so clear that a proper randomized trial cannot be ethically carried out, or occasions when the investigators have essentially no control over the allocation scheme (Kirkwood *et al.* 1997, Murray 1997). In this case, well designed non-experimental comparisons will be preferable to obtaining no information at all on the effectiveness of an intervention. As discussed by Smith and Morrow (1991, Ch. 2), non-randomized designs may also seem easier to explain to officials, to gain public acceptance, and, in general, to allow the study to be carried out in a simpler fashion, given the resistance to randomization that is often experienced. At a minimum, it seems clear that non-experimental comparisons may generate hypotheses that can subsequently be tested in a more rigorous framework. Finally, as noted by Smith *et al.* (1997), 'randomization is not a remedy for poor design, execution and analysis', i.e. it should be kept in mind that randomization alone is not a sufficient condition for sound experimentation.

The availability of a limited number of clusters is also cited as a reason to avoid randomization, since it may leave considerable imbalance between intervention groups on important prognostic factors. However, as pointed out by Koepsell *et al.* (1992), 'the difficulty of creating acceptably balanced treatment groups results chiefly from the limited number of communities available for assignment, and that difficulty remains whether randomization is used or not'. Moreover, restricted randomization, in which clusters are randomized within predefined matched pairs or strata, can be used as an alternative to simple randomization to achieve acceptable levels of balance.

A final very compelling advantage of randomized assignment is that the results are likely to have much more credibility in the scientific community, particularly if they are unexpected. This is because randomization offers the important advantage of 'a public perception of even-handedness in forming the comparison groups that is hard to achieve any other way' (Koepsell *et al.* 1992).

Reviews of studies in the health sciences have made it clear that random assignment is in fact being widely adopted to assess the effect of non-therapeutic interventions (e.g. Simpson *et al.* 1995, Smith *et al.* 1997). Similar inroads have been made in the social sciences, where Cook and Shadish (1994) suggest that successfully completed randomized trials can serve as a model in helping investigators in the social sciences to recognize that random assignment may be possible in situations where previously only quasi-experimental designs were considered. Practical issues that arise when randomization is implemented at the level of large geographic areas or organizations, where quasi-experimental designs have historically been very common, have been discussed by Ukoumunne *et al.* (1998).

In the remainder of this text, we will assume, unless otherwise stated, that the design under consideration involves random allocation.

## 1.5 The unit of inference

We mentioned in Section 1.2 that inferences in cluster randomization trials are often intended to apply at the level of the individual subject. This was arguably the case for each of the examples described in Section 1.1. However, this is not true of all cluster randomization trials. For example, consider the trial designed to evaluate the effectiveness of an intervention intended to lower the rate of caesarian section operations performed in several Latin American countries (Alexander *et al.* 1997). This study recruited 36 hospitals pair-matched on the basis of size and various geographic characteristics. The experimental intervention, consisting of solicitation of a second clinical opinion before proceeding with the operation, involves random allocation of each hospital in a matched pair. However, the target of the intervention is defined explicitly as the hospital rate of caesarian section, i.e. the trial is intended to evaluate policy at the hospital level and is not concerned with outcomes on any particular patient. Thus the hospital is the natural unit of inference in this study, and standard methods of sample size estimation and analysis would apply at the hospital level.

As a second example, consider a smoking cessation trial with communities as the unit of randomization. The target of inference in such studies could be at either the individual or community level. If the aim of the intervention was to lower the rate of smoking in a community (e.g. either by persuading individuals to cease smoking or by driving smokers out), then the community is appropriately the unit of inference. On the other hand, if the aim was specifically to influence individuals to cease smoking, then the individual is correctly seen as the appropriate unit of inference. In this case, the influence on outcome of individual-level covariates, such as a smoker's age, socioeconomic status or work history, as well as various interactions among these factors, might also be of interest.

As a final example, Kerry and Bland (1998) describe the analysis of a cluster randomization trial in which inferences are intended to apply at the general practitioner level. In this trial (Oakeshott *et al.* 1994), 34 medical practices were randomized into two groups. The practices in the experimental group received written guidelines for radiological referral adapted for general practitioners, while the control group practices received no extra guidelines. The defined outcome measure for the trial was the percentage of X-ray examinations requested that conformed to the guidelines. Thus, inferences concerning the effect of intervention were presumably intended to apply at the level of the practice rather than at the level of the individual patient.

These examples show the importance of investigators explicitly formulating and stating the hypotheses under test in cluster randomization trials. Of course, this is common-sense advice which may be said to apply to the sound planning of any comparative trial. However, the inherent ambiguity that frequently characterizes the unit of inference only adds to the value of this advice in the design of trials which randomize intact clusters of individuals. Further issues involving the unit of inference are discussed in Chapter 3 as they pertain to study planning, and in Chapters 6–8 as they pertain to data analysis.

## 1.6 Terminology: what's in a name?

In this chapter we have provided examples showing that cluster randomization designs have been adopted by health researchers in a wide range of settings. One consequence of this diversity has been that a number of essentially synonymous terms have appeared in the resulting literature.

Probably the most popular synonyms for cluster randomization are 'group randomization' and 'group allocation' (e.g. Pollock 1966, Cornfield 1978, Friedman *et al.* 1996, Pocock 1996, Murray 1998). The terms 'community randomization' or 'community intervention' trials are also often used as synonyms for cluster randomization. This may be, in part, because, as pointed out by Koepsell (1998), many of the methodological issues involved in community trials 'stem from the group-allocation feature and do not depend strongly on group size, so that similar principles apply to studies that allocate families, schools, workplaces, towns, states, nations or other social groups'. We also note that the *Dictionary of Epidemiology* (Last 1995), while omitting any reference to cluster randomization, does describe community trials as 'experiments in which the unit of allocation ... is an entire community or political subdivision'. Cluster randomization trials have also been described as macro experiments (Harris 1985) and as examples of field or social experiments (e.g. Hilton and Lumsdaine 1975, Boruch *et al.* 1978, Cook and Shadish 1994). The term 'pseudo-replication' is also closely related to the concept of clustering, since it has been used to describe the pitfall that arises when units of measurements are not independent replicates, e.g. when patients in a clinic tend to have similar outcomes (e.g. Dunn 1994).

It is also interesting to note that methodological concerns related to cluster randomization have sometimes been described as problems in defining the sampling/experimental unit (e.g. Andersen 1990, Ch. 13). Our hope is that over time the use of the term cluster randomization will predominate. This expression, we believe, more accurately reflects the study design while also reflecting the close relationship to cluster sampling.

An additional factor complicating terminology is that dependencies among responses of study subjects are not necessarily limited to cluster randomization trials or to complex surveys. Consider, for example, the individually randomized trial of HIV risk-reduction interventions reported by Jemmott *et al.* (1998). These behavioural interventions were administered by facilitators to randomly constructed 'classes' of six to eight adolescents. Responses of subjects assigned to the same class may be correlated, reflecting the personal interactions among adolescents as well as possible between-cluster variation in facilitator effects (e.g. Hopkins 1982). Similar clustering effects could arise in other individually randomized trials in which the intervention is applied on a group basis (e.g. Neuhauser and Green 1998). While we do not consider this form of clustering further, it is worth noting that the methods presented in the following chapters remain applicable to such studies.

The Medline database (Greenhalgh 1997) classifies articles dealing with cluster randomization under the MeSH (medical subject heading) of 'cluster analysis'. Articles describing complex surveys using cluster sampling (e.g. Miller and Plant 1996), those which describe methods for detecting familial, spatial or temporal clusters of disease (e.g. Alexander and Boyle 1996) and those which discuss techniques used to group variables or observations into interrelated subgroups (e.g. Everitt 1995) are all similarly classified. This common classification can prove confusing since these methods are only indirectly related to each other.

The statistical issues raised by clustering have long been recognized in the survey research field (e.g. Hansen and Hurwitz 1942, Kish 1965). Surveys differ from cluster randomization trials in that they usually involve the random selection of clusters from a defined population, but without random allocation of these clusters to different intervention groups. That is, surveys tend to be observational in nature, while cluster randomization trials are experimental. In addition, the main emphasis in surveys is on external validity, or generalizability, while in cluster randomization trials the main emphasis is generally on internal validity, i.e. on obtaining an unbiased evaluation of the intervention. This is natural since the clusters participating in such trials are rarely drawn as a random sample from a defined population. The selection of clusters participating in a survey, on the other hand, is often based on formal probabilistic considerations, with the estimation of underlying population characteristics being of primary importance. In spite of these differences, there are many analytic issues that are common to the two fields, as will be made apparent in the chapters to come.

Dependencies among cluster members are usually not of primary interest in either cluster randomization trials or complex surveys. However, the validity of statistically based conclusions is only assured when these dependencies are adjusted for in the study design and in the data analysis. These studies also are distinct from investigations which are designed specifically to detect clusters of disease, since the primary goal is then to assess factors which can explain such dependencies. For example, Conway *et al.* (1995) report on the results from a study designed to assess the household aggregation of parasitic infection by *Strongyloides stercoralis*. A key goal of this study was to determine the degree to which household aggregation was a consequence of shared risk factors, or, alternatively, of genetic predisposition to infection or possibly close contact with an infected person.

A further complication of studies investigating disease clustering is that the number and composition of the clusters might need to be determined during the investigation. This is particularly common during the investigation of temporal or geographic clusters of disease (Alexander and Boyle 1996). In cluster randomization trials, on the other hand, the number and composition of the clusters are usually known at the design stage.

The term 'cluster analysis' has also been given to methods used to place individuals into common groups or clusters as suggested by the data. For example, Peacock *et al.* (1995) used cluster analysis to identify groups of women with common sets of risk factors for having preterm babies. Three subgroups of women were identified and distinguished by maternal age and social status. As a second example, Groves *et al.* (1987) used factor analysis as well as cluster analysis to aggregate countries both by their cancer risk factor profiles and by site-specific cancer mortality rates, an analysis which led to the identification of seven distinct groups of countries.

We omit further discussion of this topic here since it is not directly relevant to the design and analysis of cluster randomization trials. Additional information may be found in standard textbooks (e.g. Everitt 1993).

# 2

# The historical development of cluster randomized trials

It has been often noted that a scientific discovery originally credited to a single individual is revealed to have been independently identified by previous investigators. This phenomenon is also well known in the statistical sciences, as pointed out by Stigler (1980). A classic example is the two-sample Wilcoxon rank sum test which has been independently proposed on at least seven different occasions (Kruskal 1957).

A similar phenomenon has characterized the historical development of cluster randomization trials. The unique analytic challenges of cluster randomization have been described independently in a number of disciplines, including educational research, teratology, the social sciences and medicine. Almost invariably, however, the actual use of this design in a given discipline has preceded investigators' recognition of the associated analytic implications. In this chapter we discuss the historical development of cluster randomization in health research, placing this development in the context of its parallel growth in other disciplines.

Section 2.1 gives an introduction to the use of random assignment in research prior to publication of the landmark randomized clinical trials conducted by the British Medical Research Council in the late 1940s. Section 2.2 provides a detailed description of cluster randomized trials conducted between 1950 and 1978. In August of 1978, the *American Journal of Epidemiology* published papers from a symposium on coronary heart disease trials (Hulley 1978). This series of articles was particularly successful in focusing attention on some of the methodological challenges unique to cluster randomization. More recent uses of cluster randomization and continuing challenges are summarized in Section 2.3. Material presented in this chapter is an extension of Section 2 from Donner and Klar (1994a).

## 2.1 Randomized trials before 1950

The use of random assignment to prevent conscious or unconscious bias in experimentation is not a recent development. Stigler (1986, Ch. 7) describes a series of experiments conducted by psychologists in the nineteenth century to determine whether there exists a minimally perceptible difference in physical stimuli. One approach used to answer this question was to determine the proportion of times that subjects could correctly state which one of two presented objects was the heavier. Peirce and Jastrow (1885) improved upon earlier experiments by offering the weights in a blinded, random sequence so that 'any possible psychological guessing of what change the operator was likely to select was avoided'. This use of random assignment is, perhaps not coincidentally, quite similar in spirit to a psychophysics example used by Fisher (1935, Ch. 2) to illustrate the principles of experimental design (Hacking 1988).

Other early uses of random assignment are discussed by McCall (1923, Ch. 3) in the context of educational research, where it is introduced as the optimal method for ensuring equivalence between experimental groups. Problems of ensuring equivalence using alternate allocation are discussed, noting, however, that 'any device which will make the selection truly random is satisfactory'. The same methods of treatment allocation recommended for students are also advocated for classrooms.

There are also several early examples of investigators recognizing the benefit of random assignment in medical research. For example, in 1648 Van Helmont suggested using assignment by lot to assess the efficacy of bloodletting for the treatment of fevers (Bloom 1986). According to Van Helmont's plan, several hundred people with fevers would first be divided into two groups. Through the casting of lots, all of the subjects in one group would be randomly assigned either to bloodletting or to a control group. Since the unit of randomization is a group of individuals, Van Helmont's trial is perhaps an early example of cluster randomization.

This trial cannot, however, be recognized as a satisfactory example of randomization since there was no replication (Armitage 1982). As will be discussed further in Chapter 3, the absence of replication completely confounds the effect of intervention with the natural variation between experimental units. A similar reservation was noted by Armitage (1972) when discussing the trial reported by Amberson *et al.* (1931). These investigators, after dividing 24 patients into two groups of 12, used a single coin flip to randomly assign all patients in a group to receive either an experimental or a control treatment. Adoption of pair-matching to create comparable groups of patients and the subsequent use of a single coin flip to assign intervention was also recommended by Hinshaw and Feldman (1944) as a useful method for conducting clinical trials.

Most other early examples of controlled trials in medicine used or advocated alternate allocation rather than random assignment (e.g. Pearson 1904, Armitage 1982). However, careful examination of the few controlled trials which report the use of random assignment suggests that this claim may be exaggerated (e.g. Houston 1991, Waller 1997). Waller (1997), for example, provides evidence suggesting that alternate assignment rather than random assignment was used in a trial of vaccines for the common cold (Diehl *et al.* 1938).

Inadequate description of treatment allocation is an ongoing problem. Williams and Davis (1994), for example, reviewed 200 clinical trials conducted in the 1980s. Of these, less than 10 per cent provided sufficient information to allow reproduction of the treatment assignment.

It should not be surprising that early investigators were largely unaware of the benefits offered by random assignment. Wide appreciation of the benefits of randomization only appeared after the publication of R. A. Fisher's (1926) paper on the arrangement of field experiments in agriculture. Speed (1991) briefly traces the impact of this work, which culminated in the publication in 1935 of Fisher's *The Design of Experiments*. A key point raised by Fisher was that valid inferences concerning the effect of intervention can only be assured when treatments are randomly assigned to replicate observations.

Fisher's work was conducted at a time of rapid growth in statistical theory. Advances made by Fisher regarding the advantages of random assignment in experimental design were matched by similar and independent descriptions of the advantages of random sampling in surveys (e.g. Neyman 1934, Rao and Bellhouse 1990). Many of the most commonly used statistical techniques (e.g. analysis of variance, Fisher's exact test, two sample and paired *t*-tests) and much of modern statistical theory were also developed during the 1920s and 1930s (see, e.g., Pearson 1966, Fienberg and Hinkley 1978).

Most medical researchers were probably not aware of these methodological advances, but if so, were largely indifferent to them. Repeated attempts to describe the value of statistical reasoning for physicians (e.g. Kilgore 1920, Mainland 1934, 1936) had only a modest impact (Marks, 1997, Ch. 5). More influential, perhaps, were Bradford Hill's series of articles on the application of statistical methods for medical research which were published in *The Lancet* in 1937 (Editor 1937, Matthews 1995, Ch. 5). Hill deliberately limited the discussion of treatment assignment to schemes involving alternate allocation, regarding these as easier to understand and less controversial than random assignment (see also Hill 1990, Silverman and Chalmers 1992).

The British Medical Research Council's 1946 study of streptomycin for the treatment of tuberculosis is generally considered to be the first publication of a clinical trial with a properly randomized control group (Medical Research Council 1948, Pocock 1983, pp. 17–18). Patients in this trial were randomly assigned either to bed rest or to bed rest plus streptomycin. Hill (1990) recounts that the decision to randomly assign patients was reached both as the fairest way to apportion the then limited supplies of streptomycin and because Hill was convinced that random assignment would ensure construction of a proper control group. The streptomycin trial stands apart because of the care taken in its design and analysis, the influence of Bradford Hill (Silverman and Chalmers 1992) and, in the long run, the success of streptomycin in treating tuberculosis (D'Arcy Hart 1972).

## 2.2 Cluster randomized trials between 1950 and 1978

The success of the streptomycin trial in instilling the virtues of random assignment among clinical researchers was at first quite modest. For example, none of the 29 clinical trials reported in the *New England Journal of Medicine* in 1953 used randomized controls (Chalmers and Schroeder 1979). In spite of a fairly steady and dramatic increase, only 50 per cent of clinical trials published in the late 1970s could claim to have employed randomization. The parallel history of randomized controlled trials for the evaluation of social programmes and public policy in the United States is discussed by Oakley (1998).

The development of methodological rigour in the design and analysis of cluster randomization trials has, in general, been substantially slower than it has been for trials randomizing individuals. This notable lag is probably due, at least in part, to the added design and analysis requirements that result from the dependencies among responses in the same cluster. However, the statistical implications of cluster randomization trials were anticipated by Lindquist (1940), who prepared a text for educational researchers based on his interpretation of Fisher's (1935) *The Design of Experiments*. This was natural since educational researchers often evaluate new methods of instruction using the classroom as the unit of randomization. Lindquist suggested that the effect of such interventions can be tested using standard statistical methods applied to cluster means. His ideas were not initially well received (McNemar 1940, Glass and Stanley 1970, pp. 501–509), with researchers in this field still debating the need to account for the effects of clustering 40 years later (e.g. Hopkins 1982, Barcikowski 1981).

There were few comparable attempts in the medical literature to distinguish randomized trials based on the unit of randomization. One notable exception was provided by Mainland (1952, pp. 114–115), who warns, in a textbook written for medical researchers, of the greater imprecision of cluster randomization, arguing that this design 'should be avoided where possible'. However, he also acknowledges that at times such trials may provide the only means of assessing the effectiveness of an intervention. His discussion is illustrated using a hospital randomized trial in which a medication for the treatment of infection by amoebiasis is assessed. The outcome in this trial was the absence of infection with the protozoan *Entamoeba histolytica* four months after treatment. Hospitals were selected as the unit of randomization because if 'in the same building, some patients had been treated and others not, the benefit of the drug might easily have been obscured by reinfection from untreated patients'. A cluster-level analysis was alluded to as an appropriate method for assessing the effect of intervention.

Many similarities exist between methodological challenges posed by cluster randomization and cluster sampling. However, the near absence of attention given to the methodological challenges posed by cluster randomized trials stands in stark contrast to the early interest expressed by statisticians in cluster sampling. For instance, Hansen and Hurwitz (1942) derived the variance for a sample proportion when the sampled unit is a cluster. The variance inflation factor obtained is identical to that shown in equation (1.1). These authors also pointed out that the increase in variance due to clustering can be quite substantial for large clusters even when the intracluster correlation coefficient is small. This phenomenon arises, they explained, because the variance inflation due to clustering is a function of both cluster size and the size of the intracluster correlation coefficient, but also because the intracluster correlation coefficient tends to decline with increasing cluster size, but at a rate that is slower than linear. A similar discussion in the context of public health surveys was provided by Cornfield (1951).

This early discussion of methods for the analyses of correlated binary data was not limited to complex surveys. Cochran (1943), for example, discusses a more general application of weighted least squares in this context, while Finney (1947, p. 60) suggests a related adjustment using probit analysis. Both approaches are early examples of methods described by Marubini *et al.* (1988) and Williams (1982), respectively.

There are very few examples of properly designed and analysed cluster randomized trials conducted by health care researchers prior to 1978. However, there were some notable exceptions conducted by epidemiologists interested in infectious disease. The methodological sophistication of these investigators is demonstrated by three double-blind, placebo-controlled trials of isoniazid (Comstock 1962, Ferebee *et al.* 1963, Horwitz and Magnus 1974), a drug used to prevent and treat tuberculosis (Berkow 1992, pp. 140–145).

In the trial reported by Ferebee *et al.* (1963), 566 hospital wards were combined into 433 units to which medication was randomly assigned. These combined wards were selected as the unit of randomization in order to reduce the administrative complexity of the trial, which involved approximately 28 000 patients. The test of intervention effect was adjusted for clustering by adapting a method described by Cochran (1953) for the analysis of sample survey data.

Many of the lessons learned by these investigators can be found in Pollock's (1966) guide to the organization and evaluation of trials of prophylactic agents for the control of communicable diseases. Careful attention is given in this guide to reasons for selecting the unit of randomization, with the implicit recognition that trials randomizing clusters are less likely to be balanced for important prognostic variables than are trials randomizing independent individuals. Reasons for randomizing clusters, as cited by Pollock (1966), included administrative convenience, reducing the risk of treatment contamination and increasing the likelihood of subject participation. It is interesting to note that very similar reasons for adopting this design were cited by Simpson *et al.* (1995) in their review of primary prevention trials published between 1990 and 1993.

The Taichung experiment (Berelson and Freedman 1964, Freedman and Takeshita 1969) is another noteworthy example of an early cluster randomized trial conducted by public health researchers. The purpose of this study, conducted between 1963 and 1965 in Taichung, Taiwan, was to assess the impact of fertility planning programmes. Taichung was then composed of approximately 2400 neighbourhood units (lins), each including about 20 households. These lins were randomly assigned to one of three experimental groups or to a control group, where the experimental groups were distinguished by the method used to convey information about birth control: (i) through the mail; (ii) by personal contact with women only; or (iii) by personal contact with both men and women. Random assignment was also stratified by population density in each of three sectors of Taichung, partly to determine whether there was any difference in the diffusion of knowledge concerning contraception in different parts of the city. The sophistication shown in this design was matched by a similar sophistication in the analysis, with the investigators clearly aware of the need to account for the effect of clustering (Freedman and Takeshita 1969, pp. 387–389).

Health care research prior to the 1950s was primarily concerned with the control and treatment of infectious diseases. However, attention slowly shifted to chronic diseases following the epidemic transition (Susser 1985). In the United States, for example, these shifting interests resulted in the growth of research into the prevention and treatment of cancer (Pocock 1983, Section 2.3) and heart disease (Hulley 1978).

Interest in lifestyle interventions for the prevention of heart disease led to the development of several community intervention trials. The two earliest were the North Karelia Project in Finland (Tuomilehto *et al.* 1980) and the Stanford Three Community Study in California (Farquhar *et al.* 1977). In the Finnish study,

North Karelia received a community-based programme to improve awareness and control of hypertension as compared with a reference community. The primary study endpoints were prevalence of hypertension and blood pressure, and measures of knowledge concerning cardiovascular risk factors. Assessments were made on approximately 5000 randomly selected subjects in each of the two communities both at baseline and after five years.

Two of the three communities in the California study were assigned to mass media campaigns designed to provide education for cardiovascular health. The mass media campaign in one of the intervention communities was supplemented with counselling for selected high-risk subjects. A third community served as a control group. Between 600 and 900 subjects were randomly sampled from each of the three communities at the start of the study. Study subjects were interviewed at baseline and 2 years later to assess knowledge and behaviour that might be related to cardiovascular disease (e.g. diet and smoking) as well as to measure blood pressure, weight and cholesterol levels.

Several reasons were given by Farquhar (1978) for omitting random assignment and enrolling only one community in each intervention group of the Stanford Three Community Study. Of these, the most important were the economic and administrative demands peculiar to community intervention trials and the need to ensure external validity, albeit at the possible cost of internal validity.

These two trials demonstrated the possibility of addressing behaviour and risk factors at the community level. Their success led to the development of similar studies in a number of different countries (Fortmann *et al.* 1995). At the same time, it was recognized that trials of lifestyle interventions inevitably involve methodological challenges different from those faced by trials designed to evaluate drugs, vaccines or surgical procedures.

These growing concerns were addressed in a symposium held at the 1977 Annual Meeting of the Society for Epidemiologic Research and published in the *American Journal of Epidemiology* (Hulley 1978). Of particular relevance was the paper by Cornfield (1978) which revisited the statistical issues raised by cluster randomization, as described earlier by Cornfield and Mitchell (1969).

Many of the justifications offered in this symposium for adopting cluster randomization were identical to reasons cited by Pollock (1966) for trials of prophylactic agents used in the control of communicable diseases. Indeed, in commenting on the symposium, Comstock (1978) noted, with some regret, that the lessons learned by tuberculosis researchers did not appear to be widely recognized among investigators in other disciplines.

These concerns, although well founded, were gradually being addressed in the epidemiological literature. For example, MacMahon and Pugh (1970, pp. 291–293), in their classic text on epidemiological methods, had warned investigators of the inferential limitations of trials which include only one community per intervention group. They also drew attention to the guide prepared by Pollock (1966) for investigators designing intervention trials. This discussion was extended to cancer screening trials by Apostolides and Henderson (1977), and more generally to health and medical care evaluation by Henderson and Meinert (1975).

The debate over the proper approach to the design and analysis of trials involving clustered observations was not limited to epidemiology. Similar discussions were taking place in the laboratory sciences (e.g. Weil 1970, Haseman and Hogan 1975, Williams 1975), among educational researchers (e.g. Burstein and Smith 1977) and in the social sciences (e.g. Bennett and Lumsdaine 1975). These debates and related discussions concerning repeated measurements (e.g. Ederer 1973) further spurred an interest in developing new methodology for cluster randomization trials.

## 2.3 Cluster randomized trials since 1978

As the 1980s began, medical researchers aware of the need to account for the effects of clustering had few resources to help them in the design and analysis of cluster randomized trials. This omission began gradually to be addressed as papers illustrating methods were published (e.g. Gillum *et al.* 1980, Donner *et al.* 1981).

This decade also saw a dramatic increase in the development of methods for analysing correlated outcome data, many of which could be directly applied to cluster randomized trials. The impetus for this work arose in many diverse fields, including dentistry (Imrey and Chilton 1992), ophthalmology (Rosner 1984), longitudinal studies (Ware and Liang 1996), survey sampling (Rao and Bellhouse 1990) and teratology (Krewski *et al.* 1996). Particular progress was made in the development of statistical methods for the analysis of correlated categorical data (see, e.g. Ashby *et al.* 1992).

As might be expected, publication of this work did not immediately translate into any marked improvement in the methodological quality of cluster randomized trials. The difficulties investigators continued to experience with the design and analysis of cluster randomization trials were demonstrated in several methodological reviews. Donner *et al.* (1990) reviewed 16 studies of non-therapeutic interventions published between 1979 and 1989; Simpson *et al.* (1995) limited attention to 21 primary prevention trials published in either the *American Journal of Public Health* or *Preventive Medicine* between 1990 and 1993; while Smith *et al.* (1997) identified nine cluster randomized trials as part of their more general review of community health trials published in 1992.

Similar results were reported in each of these reviews, with less than 25 per cent of the studies considered accounting for between-cluster variation when determining trial power. The situation was somewhat improved with respect to data analysis, where the effects of clustering were seen to be accounted for by at least 50 per cent of the trials considered in each review.

These dismal results are consistent with those found by Altman and Bland (1991), who after reading 150 methodological reviews of articles from medical journals reported that about half the published papers in the medical literature are statistically flawed. They also found that problems are more likely to be due to an inadequate description of design, e.g. a failure to explain how sample size was determined, rather than to a flaw in the analysis. This suggests that the methodological difficulties that characterize reports of cluster randomization trials may be no more severe than those found in other study designs.

There is even reason to be optimistic. First, there is evidence that technological advances in statistics are diffusing more rapidly in the medical literature (Altman and Goodman 1994). Second, additional and continuing attention is being given in the medical literature to the proper design and analysis of cluster randomized trials (Bland and Kerry 1997). Third, consideration of the unit of randomization and of appropriate methods of analysis and reporting are now being included in standard checklists for reporting randomized controlled trials (e.g. Begg *et al.* 1996).

# 3

# Issues arising in the planning of cluster randomization trials

Investigators planning a cluster randomization trial need to consider three issues that correspond closely to those proposed by Pocock (1983) in his discussion of therapeutic trials: (i) the choice of interventions to be evaluated; (ii) the choice of eligibility criteria, both on an individual and on a cluster level; and (iii) the assessment of subject responses. These issues, which must be addressed in all cluster randomization trials, are discussed in detail in Sections 3.1, 3.2 and 3.3, respectively.

Several different experimental designs have been specifically proposed for cluster randomization trials. Section 3.4 describes the three designs most frequently adopted, while Section 3.5 discusses some less frequently used designs. Guidelines for choosing an experimental design are provided in Sections 3.6 and 3.7, while some strategies for conducting successful cluster randomization trials are presented in Section 3.8.

## 3.1 Selecting interventions

New therapeutic agents must pass through three phases of development prior to their being made part of standard medical practice (Friedman *et al.* 1996). Phase I trials are designed to identify the appropriate dose of medication. These trials generally represent the first use of a new drug in humans. Estimates of the biological activity and rates of toxicity of the new drug are then assessed as part of a phase II trial at the dose suggested by the phase I trial. Only drugs whose biological activity and rates of toxicity are acceptable as compared with historical controls will be included in randomized comparative trials, i.e. a phase III trial. An analogous approach is typically used to identify effective chemopreventive agents (Buiatti 1996, Greenwald and Kelloff 1996).

In contrast, however, there have been few attempts to develop analogous phases for assessing health promotion programmes (Flay 1986, Cullen 1990, Brownson *et al.* 1997). The absence of such a systematic approach complicates the selection of appropriate interventions. Too early evaluation of an unproven programme is not worth the major commitment of cost and time required by a randomized trial, while random assignment of programmes already in wide use might not be feasible or even perceived as ethical. The continuing change that characterizes the communities and cultures to which these programmes are to be applied also heightens the importance of social and behavioural theory in developing viable interventions (e.g. Baranowski *et al.* 1997).

The absence of accepted guidelines for selecting interventions in health promotion trials may have unfortunate consequences by leading to the unnecessary utilization of scarce resources. It is interesting to note that four of the 16 cluster randomization trials reviewed by Donner *et al.* (1990) involved three intervention groups, while 11 of the 21 trials reviewed by Simpson *et al.* (1995) compared three or more groups. Although there is obvious merit in being able to identify the optimal intervention among several competitors, the resulting gains will not be realized if limited resources prevent a corresponding increase in the number of clusters that can be enrolled, thus reducing statistical power.

Trials of new medication are often designed using placebo controls when no proven treatment is available. These biologically inactive substances are then used to distinguish the direct effect of a new treatment from the remarkable ability of a subjective belief to cause clinically relevant improvements in health, known as the placebo effect (Ernst and Herxheimer, 1996). Placebo controls also have the advantage of facilitating the blinding of both patients and clinicians to the assigned intervention.

A number of double-blind, placebo-controlled cluster randomization trials have been conducted (e.g. Comstock 1962, Ferebee *et al.* 1963, Horwitz and Magnus 1974, West *et al.* 1991). However, control group subjects in cluster randomization trials most often receive whatever programme they would have received in the absence of the intervention, as was the case in 14 of the 21 primary prevention trials reviewed by Simpson *et al.* (1995). Observed effects of intervention could then be attributed, at least in part, to the added attention given to subjects in the experimental group, i.e. to a Hawthorne effect (Buck and Donner 1982). Rates of attrition might also vary across intervention groups as a consequence of this phenomenon. To offset the impact of these effects, two alternative control group interventions have been proposed: wait-list controls and 'minimal intervention' or 'active' controls.

Subjects in a wait-list control group receive the intervention, but only after its effect has been assessed in subjects assigned to the experimental group. This strategy was employed, for example, by Walker *et al.* (1992) in their family-based cardiovascular disease prevention trial. Adoption of a wait-list control group might encourage an equal degree of participation across groups, since all subjects would eventually receive the benefits of the intervention programme. However, it is clearly practical only for trials having a relatively short follow-up period.

An alternative in other trials may be an active control group that is perceived to be of equal value to the study participants and selected so that it will not interfere with the primary comparison of interest. This strategy was adopted, for example, by Haggerty *et al.* (1994) in their community-based hygiene educational trial for the prevention of diarrhoeal morbidity. Intervention communities received an educational programme to prevent the occurrence of diarrhoea, while control communities received education in the prevention of dehydration during diarrhoea.

Difficulties in distinguishing the effects of intervention from Hawthorne effects may also be avoided by using more than one type of control group (see Buck and Donner 1982). Adoption of two or more control groups would also permit a more accurate interpretation of dropout patterns. Unfortunately this strategy usually offers little practical benefit, given the limited number of clusters typically available to investigators. We discuss the ethical implications of choosing different types of control groups in Chapter 4.

## 3.2 Setting eligibility criteria

Therapeutic trials are often designed using quite stringent eligibility criteria to reduce between-subject variability and thereby to increase the power of the study (Yusuf *et al.* 1990, George 1996, Fuks *et al.* 1998). These restrictions are intended to limit the patient population to individuals who are likely to benefit from the intervention and to show high levels of compliance. However, in addition to complicating the study design, the use of overly restrictive criteria can have several unintended, deleterious consequences (e.g. Yusuf *et al.* 1990). The most obvious of these is that it is often more difficult to generalize results from trials which use strict eligibility criteria. The added administrative complexities involved can also limit accrual and increase the possibility of protocol violations caused by enrolling ineligible patients. The burden of added screening requirements might also increase the cost of the trial.

These considerations also apply to setting eligibility criteria for cluster randomization trials. Here, however, these criteria need to be specified at both the cluster level and the individual level. Eligibility criteria at the cluster level are, to a certain extent, determined by the selected interventions. For example, interventions which make use of mass media to influence health behaviour (e.g. COMMIT Research Group 1995a) will naturally select the community as the unit of randomization. Similarly, schools are the obvious unit of randomization for smoking cessation trials aimed at adolescents (e.g. Murray *et al.* 1992). For trials such as these, the main task is to decide how similar or heterogeneous the selected sample of clusters should be.

Given the complexity and multifaceted nature of many of the interventions evaluated in cluster randomization trials, as well as the heterogenous populations to which these interventions are often applied, it seems reasonable to characterize a large percentage of these studies as 'effectiveness' trials. Such trials have been defined (e.g. Flay 1986) as providing tests of intervention under 'real world' conditions, as opposed to efficacy trials, which provide tests of intervention under 'optimum conditions'. Thus efficacy trials would select clusters and subjects according to fairly restrictive eligibility criteria, would exhibit little variability in the manner in which the intervention is implemented, and would expect to observe fairly high levels of subject compliance. Although conditions similar to these are often seen in clinical drug trials, they are less characteristic of health research trials that randomize intact social units.

However, investigators occasionally have much greater latitude in selecting the unit of randomization. Thus trials of vitamin A supplementation on child mortality have been conducted using several different units of assignment, including individual children, households and communities (Fawzi *et al.* 1993). For these trials, the final selection of the randomization unit will inevitably represent a compromise among several factors, including statistical power, the need to ensure independence in responses among different units of randomization, the desire to avoid contamination, what is administratively most feasible, the method by which the intervention is applied, and its anticipated effect. For example, in some studies it might be prudent to randomize larger clusters such as communities if the impact of the intervention is expected to be greater when a relatively very large number of individuals are exposed, thus adding to overall 'synergy'. In statistical terms, this may be thought of as 'securing' the size of the intervention effect. Sorensen *et al.* (1998) address this issue when they stress the importance of 'contextualization', in which individual behaviours (and hence outcomes) are culturally and structurally maintained in community intervention trials.

Investigators sometimes have very direct control over the unit of randomization. This was the case, for example, in a controlled trial of nursing services intended to improve the health of individuals undergoing cardiac surgery and the functioning of their family groups (Gilliss *et al.* 1993). The experimental intervention consisted of in-hospital education and counselling for patients and the primary care-giver. Cluster randomization was adopted in order to avoid the contamination that could result if patients and their family members assembled to discuss the study. The cluster in this case was formed by taking a fixed number of consecutive patients who entered into the study at a given site. Thus the unit of randomization in this trial was not a closed, naturally formed group, as it is in most such studies, but rather was created on the basis of temporal factors. Consequently, although the number of potential sites for the trial was limited, the investigators had systematic control over the number of patients who could be entered per site.

Investigator control over cluster size may also be possible when the randomization unit consists of a selected number of geographically contiguous sites. For example, Morrow *et al.* (1999) report on a randomized controlled trial of the effectiveness of home-based peer counselling to promote exclusive breast-feeding. In this trial, clusters of two to four city blocks were randomized in order to minimize the contamination from influences expected if relatives and close neighbours were assigned to different study groups. The actual number of blocks chosen per cluster was, at least to some extent, a design choice. This type of latitude on the part of the investigators clearly provides some administrative advantages as well as increased flexibility in the means to achieve the desired trial power.

Different units of randomization may at times be included in the same trial. For example, Moore and Tsiatis (1991) describe a Russian trial of breast self-examination in which factories were the unit of randomization in Moscow, while polyclinics were the unit of randomization in Leningrad. A more ambitious scheme was described by Simon (1981), who suggested that randomization of both individuals and physicians' practices can be incorporated into a single trial. The main purpose of this design is to increase accrual to therapeutic trials when some of the recruited physicians will participate only if all of their patients receive the same intervention.

Having decided on the unit of randomization, investigators will usually specify additional cluster-level eligibility criteria. In some trials, these will be quite detailed, as in the trial of domestic water filters on gastrointestinal disease reported by Payment *et al.* (1991). In this study, participating households were randomly assigned to continue using tap water or, alternatively, to have a water filter installed. Five very specific household eligibility criteria were listed:

1. owner-occupied;
2. French-speaking occupants;
3. regular consumers of tap water (as opposed to bottled or filtered water);
4. at least one child between the ages of 2 and 18 living in the household;
5. willingness to participate in a longitudinal trial in which a random half of the households would have a filter installed.

Trials in which the unit of randomization is a family or a household typically include data from all eligible cluster members. A subsampling strategy, however, might be preferable when larger units such as communities are randomly assigned. For example, approximately 550 heavy smokers and 550 light-to-moderate smokers were identified in each of the participating COMMIT communities to assess the effect of the intervention on smoking cessation (COMMIT Research Group 1995a). Careful specification of eligibility criteria is again required, balancing concern for generalizability with the need for internal validity. The implications of subsampling for the determination of the overall sample size are discussed in Chapter 5.

It is typical of most individually randomized trials that the identity of study subjects is not known at baseline, since accrual gradually occurs over time. This complicates the ability to determine the effect of setting stringent eligibility criteria at the individual level until a sizeable proportion of the study subjects have been enrolled. However, in the case of cluster randomization trials, there are many examples in which the identities of all participating subjects are known in advance. For example, in worksite trials a census of all eligible companies is often conducted prior to random assignment (e.g. Thompson *et al.* 1997a). The known baseline characteristics of worksites and employees can then provide important information concerning generalizability at an early stage of the trial. These surveys might also provide information which could prove helpful in selecting the actual study design.

## 3.3 Measuring subject response

Decisions regarding what data to collect and how to measure subject response should be guided primarily by the study objectives. In this section we discuss related issues, including the unit of inference, the number of repeated assessments per subject or cluster, the anticipated effects of intervention and the available resources. We pay particular attention to the choice between a cohort design which tracks the same individuals over time (identified prior to random assignment) and a repeated cross-sectional design that tracks the same clusters, but draws independent samples of individuals at each time point.

Many of these issues are illustrated by the Child and Adolescent Trial for Cardiovascular Health (CATCH), first discussed in Chapter 1. Schools in this trial were randomly assigned to a school-based intervention, a combined school-based and family-based intervention, or a 'usual curriculum' control group (Zucker *et al.* 1995, Luepker *et al.* 1996). The school-based intervention included training sessions for teachers in the CATCH curricula, instruction for food service personnel in providing more nutritional school meals, and health education activities based in the classroom. These programmes were supplemented by at-home activities for those students assigned to the combined school-based and family-based intervention.

The primary objective of this trial was to compare the change in serum cholesterol from baseline to the end of the intervention period for students in the experimental group as compared with students in the control group. However, several secondary objectives were also of interest. These included the effect of intervention on the quality of food services and on self-reported diet, assessed at the level of the school and individual, respectively. The effect of the intervention on food services was determined by conducting a dietary analysis of the school lunch menus. Dietary information based on a 24-hour recall was collected at baseline and follow-up from a randomly selected cohort of students.

The identification of several distinct endpoints, some at the school level and others at the student level, offered several advantages (Feldman 1997). First, it increased the possibility of detecting distinct effects of intervention at these different levels of aggregation. Second, the typically decreased costs associated with the cluster-level endpoints (e.g. dietary analysis of school menus) as compared with the individual-level endpoints (e.g. 24-hour diet recall) served an important practical purpose. Third, cluster-level endpoints may be more objective and less prone to bias than endpoints collected from individual study subjects (see Koepsell 1998).

The CATCH was also noteworthy for the care investigators took in determining on how many occasions each endpoint was to be assessed and whether or not repeated assessments were to be made on the same or on different subjects. For instance, cholesterol measurements were taken twice: at baseline when the students were in grade three and again at the end of the intervention in grade six. Requests for blood samples used to determine cholesterol levels were limited to the cohort of students whose cholesterol levels were determined at baseline.

Plans for tracking students who transferred to another school were also incorporated into the protocol. This was deemed necessary since students who transferred might be different from those who did not, and the reasons for transferring might vary across intervention groups. Methods for tracking subjects that may help to reduce the rate of attrition and the consequent risk of bias have been discussed by Morrison *et al.* (1997) in the context of a smoking prevention cluster randomization trial. More general discussion is provided by Hunt and White (1998).

Alternative design strategies were also considered by the CATCH investigators. One possibility was to request blood draws from a sample of students attending participating schools at each assessment point. A principal attraction of such repeated cross-sectional surveys is that concerns regarding attrition would be avoided. Of course, differential rates of participation in cross-sectional surveys conducted after random assignment can still compromise validity, the principal concern being that willingness to participate may be a consequence of the intervention. Nonetheless, random samples of respondents at each assessment time may be more representative of the target population than a fixed cohort of students. For example, cohort members may differ from the target population by their willingness to participate at more than one time point. A further disadvantage of the cohort approach is that a subject's participation at a given point of assessment might affect his or her responses at a later assessment point (Holt 1989).

Studies which follow subjects for an appreciable length of time also need to consider that the increasing mean age of cohort members might hinder generalizability at the cluster level. For example, cohorts of heavy smokers were followed for four years in the COMMIT smoking cessation trial (COMMIT Research Group 1995a). However, the average age of people living in cities which participated in COMMIT might not have changed over the same time period. Migration of subjects in and out of clusters can also change their composition, particularly in studies with long follow-up times (e.g. Jooste *et al.* 1990). For all of these reasons, repeated cross-sectional surveys are most useful when inferences are directed at the cluster level.

Repeated cross-sectional surveys are less useful, however, when investigating the effect of intervention on changing the health or behaviour of individual study subjects. Under these circumstances, it is preferable to follow cohorts of subjects over time, focusing on the individual as the unit of analysis. A further advantage of the cohort approach in this case is that it allows a direct determination of the degree to which individual subjects have actually received the intervention. This approach may be particularly natural when the unit of random assignment is a family or household, since it may not be feasible in this case to obtain independent cross-sectional samples of subjects from the same cluster at each assessment point.

Decisions regarding the selection of a cohort or cross-sectional design should be based primarily on the study objectives and the associated unit of inference. However, it can still be informative to quantitatively evaluate the relative efficiency of the two designs, a task which requires that two sources of correlation between repeated assessments over time be distinguished.

In Chapter 1, the intracluster correlation coefficient was derived by considering the variation in response among clusters. In a similar fashion, temporal variation induces a correlation in the mean scores which correspond to a cluster at two different time points. This latter parameter, which may be referred to as the 'cluster-level autocorrelation', will result in some gain in power for the repeated cross-sectional survey. Any further gains in power obtained by using a cohort design may then be modest unless there is also a large degree of individual-level autocorrelation. Furthermore, subject attrition may well further reduce or even eliminate any incremental gains in power that may be obtained using a cohort design.

The joint contribution of individual-level and cluster-level autocorrelation to the efficiency of cross-sectional relative to cohort designs has been studied by Feldman and McKinlay (1994), as subsequently extended by McKinlay (1994) to incorporate costs. The impact of subject attrition on the choice between the two designs is explored in detail by Diehr *et al.* (1995a). Table 3.1 provides a summary of the factors involved in choosing one design over the other.

More sophisticated designs which combine both cross-sectional samples and cohorts of subjects in the same study have also been adopted (e.g. Diehr *et al.* 1995a). These designs allow one to assess the degree to which cohort members are distinct from subjects asked to participate at only one time point. Differences can then be explored between subjects who remain in the cluster throughout the entire study and subjects who migrate in or out. However, the enrolment of both cross-sectional samples and cohorts of subjects should only be considered after the investigators are assured that there is sufficient power to attain the primary study objectives.

**Table 3.1** Factors affecting the selection of cohort versus cross-sectional designs (Feldman and McKinlay 1994)

| | |
|---|---|
| 1. | Study objectives |
| 2. | Unit of inference |
| 3. | Cluster size |
| 4. | Statistical efficiency |
| 5. | Rate of attrition |
| 6. | Length of trial |
| 7. | Population stability |
| 8. | Number of assessments |
| 9. | Effect of measurement |
| 10. | Effect of intervention |

We note, in concluding this section, that it is important to provide some justification for the number and timing of each of the specified assessments. Most studies will include a baseline assessment. The data resulting from this assessment can help to assess the effectiveness of the randomization in creating balance, may be used to improve precision in testing the effect of intervention, and may be useful in achieving secondary objectives concerning the effect of selected risk factors on outcome. In studies where all available clusters are enrolled simultaneously, baseline data may also be used to help identify potential stratification variables.

The number and timing of assessments made after baseline should be determined by the anticipated temporal responses in each intervention group. Koepsell *et al.* (1991) consider several different time trends which could occur when comparing responses of subjects from clusters assigned to an intervention group with responses of subjects from clusters assigned to a control group. For example, it might be reasonable to expect different linear trends over time in a community randomized trial of a peer education programme for smoking prevention if the effects of intervention were expected to diffuse slowly through each community. Conversely, the effects of intervention might diffuse rapidly but be transient, requiring a more careful determination of assessment times so that the effect is not missed. Theoretical models that might prove helpful in selecting relevant variables and their assessment times are discussed by Baranowski *et al.* (1997) in the context of behavioural studies.

## 3.4 The most commonly used experimental designs

There are three designs that are most frequently adopted in cluster randomization trials:

- completely randomized, involving no pre-stratification or matching of clusters according to baseline characteristics;
- matched-pair, in which one of two clusters in a stratum are randomly assigned to each intervention;
- stratified, involving the assignment of two or more clusters to at least some combinations of stratum and intervention.

An interesting example of the completely randomized design is given by the ACEH study, as reported by Abdeljaber *et al.* (1991). This trial was designed to evaluate the effectiveness of vitamin A supplementation on symptoms of respiratory and enteric infections among Indonesian children aged one to five years. The primary outcome variable was the one-year prevalence of cough, fever and diarrhoea, with villages adopted as the unit of randomization.

The completely randomized design is most suited to trials randomizing a fairly large number of clusters, as in the example above where 229 villages were assigned to the experimental group and 221 to the control. This was also the case in the vitamin A trial conducted by Sommer *et al.* (1986), discussed earlier in Chapter 1. Otherwise, however, some matching or stratification in the design is usually advisable. This is because of the well-accepted design principle (e.g. Pocock 1983, Section 5.3) that stratification is most effective in small studies, a principle which is particularly relevant to cluster randomization trials, where the effective sample size may be much less than the actual number of individuals enrolled. As in all clinical trials, however, it is only worthwhile to stratify on cluster-level factors known to be strongly associated with outcome.

One stratification factor frequently adopted by investigators is cluster size, as grouped into categories such as small, medium and large. This is a particularly attractive choice if it is believed that the size of a cluster may act as a surrogate for within-cluster dynamics that are predictive of outcome, or otherwise may be associated with important cluster-level factors. For example, if the size of a school is thought to affect academic performance, size then becomes a natural matching factor in the design of school-based intervention studies. Stratification by cluster size may also increase efficiency in that it assures approximately the same number of subjects in each arm of the trial. For the comparison of means using *t*-tests or the analysis of variance, equal sample sizes are also advantageous in that they lead to greater robustness with respect to moderate departures from the underlying assumptions of normality and homogeneity of variance (Miller 1997, Section 2.3). Other stratification factors that are frequently adopted in cluster randomization trials include geographic area, categorized levels of baseline event rates and macro-level measures of socioeconomic status. An interesting example of how failure to stratify on socioeconomic status led to serious interpretational difficulties in a breast cancer screening trial randomizing medical practices is given by Alexander *et al.* (1989).

The matched-pair design has been widely used in community intervention trials. The main advantage of this design is its potential to provide very tight and explicit balancing of potentially important prognostic factors at baseline. This may enhance the perceived credibility of the trial conclusions. An illustrative example is the COMMIT trial, designed to promote smoking cessation using a variety of community resources (COMMIT Research Group 1995a). The primary outcome variable for this trial was the five year smoking cessation rate among heavy smokers. The design involved 11 pairs of communities matched on the basis of community size, population density, demographic profile, community structure and geographical proximity.

The ability of the matched-pair design to create intervention groups that are perceived to be comparable at baseline requires a consensus as to which potential matching factors are the most important. This point was noted by Sanson-Fisher *et al.* (1996), who stated that 'unless a matched pair (of clusters) somewhat appear to be similar, it is unlikely that the results of the research will be accepted as valid'. Prognostically important differences can, as an alternative to matching, be adjusted for in the statistical analysis. As pointed out by Smith and Morrow (1991), however, a possible counterbalancing factor is that 'the persuasiveness of the results may be reduced if the conclusions depend upon extensive statistical manipulation'.

In spite of its obvious abilities for creating comparable groups of subjects, there are some analytic limitations of this design that have received attention in the context of community intervention trials (Martin *et al.* 1993, Klar and Donner 1997). These limitations arise largely from the practical difficulty of obtaining close matches on important prognostic factors and from the difficulty in estimating the intracluster correlation from matched-pair data. These issues are further discussed in Section 3.6.

The stratified design is an extension of the matched-pair design in which several clusters, rather than just one, are randomly assigned within strata to each of the intervention and control groups. An example of this design is provided by CATCH, discussed most recently in Section 3.3. In this study the unit of randomization was the elementary school, with each school contributing approximately 53 grade three students. The strata consisted of four cities in the United States, with 24 schools randomly assigned to the experimental or control group within each city.

In some trials, the choice of stratification variables may be dictated as much by practical as by scientific considerations. For example, in order to obtain the cooperation of investigators in a school-based trial, it may be necessary to stratify by school district in order to reassure administrators that at least some schools in each district will receive the experimental intervention.

The use of restricted randomization to create balance on important baseline covariates is admittedly possible only when the number of clusters is reasonably large relative to the number of potential stratification variables. When the number of clusters is limited, but several potential confounding variables have been identified, it may be impossible to match or stratify by all these variables individually. For this type of situation, Graham *et al.* (1984) have proposed a 'multiattribute utility measurement (MAUM) approach'. After identifying a set of relatively uncorrelated potential confounders (e.g. using factor analysis), the variables are combined so as to yield a single score for each cluster. Subject to the assumption that the original variables are additive, this score may then be categorized and used as a matching factor to help reduce group differences on all variables simultaneously. Interested readers might wish to consult the related literature on propensity score methods, as proposed for defining strata in matched case–control or cohort studies (e.g. Joffe and Rosenbaum 1999).

Most often, clusters are randomized within strata that may be regarded as fixed. For example, this will almost certainly be the case when strata are defined using the previously described MAUM approach. Thompson *et al.* (1997b), however, discuss a matched-pair trial in which two general medical practices were selected from a representative sample of British towns, thus allowing differences among towns to be regarded as a random effect. Inferences in this case could reasonably be directed to the population of all British towns on the basis of sampling considerations. For the fixed-effects approach, on the other hand, inferences intended to apply beyond the strata represented in the study must be based on judgment and previous knowledge of between-stratum heterogeneity.

Many of the same issues have arisen in the ongoing controversy regarding the relative advantages of these two approaches in the meta-analyses of individually randomized trials (e.g. see Fleiss 1993). However, given the paucity of this research as applied to the design and analysis of cluster randomization trials, we limit our attention, unless stated otherwise, to the fixed-effects approach.

## 3.5 Factorial and crossover designs

We have limited attention in the previous sections to experimental designs in which study participants are exposed to only one of the interventions being evaluated. In this section we consider more complex factorial and crossover designs. A common feature of both designs is that study participants may be exposed to more than one of the interventions being evaluated. Moreover, both designs have been recommended based on their potential for increasing power (e.g. Piantadosi 1997, Chs 15–16). However, it should be recognized that any potential gains in power are realized only when fairly stringent assumptions are satisfied, limiting the usefulness of these designs as applied to cluster randomization trials.

The trial of interventions for the prevention of low back pain, reported by van Poppel *et al.* (1998), illustrates the simplest application of a factorial design. This trial was conducted among cargo department workers of an airline located in the Netherlands. A total of 36 work groups, each consisting of six to 20 workers, were randomized to one of four intervention groups: (1) education (lifting instructions) and lumbar support, (2) education alone, (3) lumbar support alone, and (4) no intervention. The main outcomes were the prevalence and duration of low back pain and sick leave. Technically this is known as a $2 \times 2$ factorial design (e.g. Fleiss 1986, Ch. 12), since each of the two interventions was assigned at one of two levels, i.e. education (yes/no) and lumbar support (yes/no). More complicated factorial designs including more than two factors and/or allowing for three or more levels of a factor have also been used, at least for individually randomized clinical trials (Piantadosi 1997, p. 397).

It is clear why factorial designs are attractive in principle. Suppose, for example, there was reason to believe in the trial described above that education and lumbar support act independently to prevent low back pain, i.e. it could be assumed that there is no interaction between these two factors. Then the same subjects could be used to estimate the separate effects on back pain prevention of both lumbar support and education. Estimates of each intervention effect could be calculated with the same degree of precision that would be obtained if the trial were restricted to an investigation of that factor alone.

Unfortunately investigators will rarely be able to rule out the possibility of interaction between interventions. For example, the effect of lumbar support might vary depending on whether or not subjects also received lifting instructions. Indeed the opportunity to examine the joint effects of two or more interventions is a primary advantage of factorial trials. However, this advantage will only be fully realized if there is sufficient power to detect interaction effects, which in turn will require a much larger trial than one designed to detect main effects only. Concern for misguided assumptions that interventions act independently in studies which have insufficient power to properly evaluate interaction effects prompted Lubsen and Pocock (1994) to note that in factorial trials 'the numbers may look bigger than they really are'.

Notwithstanding these concerns, adequately powered factorial designs can prove particularly useful for trials of health education interventions. Kvalem *et al.* (1996), for example, randomly assigned 124 classrooms either to a school-based sex education programme or to a control group. Classrooms were also randomly assigned to receive either a baseline assessment and a follow-up assessment or only a follow-up assessment. The primary study outcomes were students' sexual behaviour at six months and one year after the introduction of the intervention. This design was selected, at least in part, to distinguish the effect of intervention from any effect induced by the baseline assessment itself, i.e. from a version of the Hawthorne effect. It is interesting to note that similar designs were discussed much earlier by Campbell and Stanley (1963, pp. 24–26).

Economic and administrative difficulties in recruiting a sufficient number of clusters to adequately assess interaction effects can be lessened somewhat if it is feasible for one of the factors to be randomly assigned at the individual level. Thus Marbiah *et al.* (1998) report on a factorial trial of malarial control interventions in which 17 pair-matched villages were randomly assigned to receive either insecticide-impregnated bed nets or no nets. Children within each village were then individually randomized to either chemoprophylaxis or placebo. Additional discussion of this design, also known as a split-plot design, is provided by Fleiss (1986, Ch. 13) in the context of clinical experimentation.

Participants in factorial trials are typically assigned to all intervention arms simultaneously. This is to be distinguished from a crossover design where participants receive two or more interventions in a randomly determined order, thus removing between-subject variability from the intervention comparison (Friedman *et al.* 1996, Ch. 4). This design also ensures that each cluster enrolled in the trial receives each intervention, thus alleviating ethical concerns that might otherwise arise. However, the validity of the crossover design depends on the assumption that carry-over effects are absent, i.e. that the estimated effects of intervention are independent of the order in which they were assigned. This issue seriously complicated the interpretation of an early application of the crossover design to a hospital intervention trial (Turpeinen *et al.* 1979). The effect of diet on heart disease was examined in this trial by assigning a cholesterol-lowering diet or a standard diet to all patients in one of two psychiatric hospitals in Finland. The hospitals switched meal plans after six years. However, since mortality was the primary outcome, any patient who participated in the entire trial would be a highly selected survivor (Halperin *et al.* 1973). More recent applications of crossover designs have been reported by Palmer *et al.* (1985) in their study of quality assurance in 16 ambulatory care practices and by Menzies *et al.* (1993) in their study of 'sick building syndrome'. In all such applications, the estimated effect of intervention may be biased in the presence of carry-over effects.

There are several additional administrative complications that apply to both factorial and crossover designs when these are adopted for cluster randomization trials. Compliance might be difficult to ensure, for example, in those arms of a factorial design in which clusters are required to receive more than one intervention. It might be even more difficult to expect a uniformly timed replacement of one intervention by another, as would be required for a crossover trial.

The combination of statistical and practical concerns associated with these designs suggests that investigators planning cluster randomization trials should use caution before rejecting the possibility of adopting less complicated methods of evaluation. We therefore omit any further discussion of factorial or crossover designs in this chapter.

## 3.6 Selecting an experimental design

The purpose of pair-matching in the design stage of a cluster randomization trial is to reduce imbalance on baseline risk factors, thus improving the power for detecting intervention effects as well as increasing the credibility or face validity of the trial. In this section we explore in more detail the strengths and weaknesses of this design as compared with other designs that could be adopted.

The power of the matched-pair design as compared with that of the completely randomized design will gradually improve as the effectiveness of the matching increases. The increase in efficiency induced by the matching will depend directly on the size of the matching correlation $\rho_M$, a parameter to be distinguished from the intracluster correlation coefficient $\rho$ discussed in Chapter 1. The matching correlation $\rho_M$ may be regarded as the standard Pearson correlation as computed over the paired clusters. The relative efficiency of the matched-pair design as compared with the completely randomized design (ignoring differences in degrees of freedom) is given by $1/(1-\rho_M)$. Details of the derivation are provided by Donner (1998) and Freedman *et al.* (1997) in the context of binary outcome data, while Shipley *et al.* (1989) describe analogous gains in efficiency for incidence rate data. Arguments provided by Freedman *et al.* (1997) are also directly applicable to analyses of quantitative outcomes. These expressions show, as might be expected, that the effectiveness of matching depends on the ability of the investigator to create pairs of clusters (strata) that vary as much as possible with respect to baseline risk. However, these calculations do not take into account that there are half as many effective observations to estimate the variance in a matched design as there are in an unmatched design. Martin *et al.* (1993), by taking into account this factor, arrived at a more accurate comparison of statistical power between the two designs for the case of a small to moderate number of pair-matched clusters. A principal conclusion from this comparison was that if the number of available pairs is 10 or less, matching should be used only if the value of $\rho_M$ is at least 0.20, a conclusion which is consistent with the known relationship between the critical values for Student's *t*-test and its degrees of freedom. This relationship was examined in detail by Festing (1996), who showed that the minimum size of intervention effect that can be detected at $\alpha = 0.05$ begins to increase very rapidly as the degrees of freedom fall from about 10 to 2. Thus for very small studies, involving less than six matched pairs, extremely high correlations are needed for matching to be effective. Martin *et al.* (1993) therefore remarked that 'it is unlikely that effective matching would be possible for small studies. Matching may be overused as a design tool.'

This discussion raises the question of what values of $\rho_M$ tend to occur in practice. Table 3.2 reports values of this parameter as estimated empirically from data arising from seven matched-pair trials published since 1987. The magnitude of the computed

**Table 3.2** Values of estimated matching correlations in matched-pair trials

| Source | Unit of randomization | Number of pairs | Outcome variable | Matching correlation |
|---|---|---|---|---|
| Stanton & Clemens (1987) | Cluster of families | 25 | Childhood rate of diarrhoea | 0.49 |
| Bass *et al.* (1986) | Physician practice | 17 | Death rate | 0.41 |
| Thompson *et al.* (1997b) | Physician practice | 13 | Levels of coronary risk factors | 0.13 |
| Ray *et al.* (1997) | Nursing home | 7 | Rate of recurrent falling | 0.63 |
| Haggerty *et al.* (1994) | Community | 9 | Childhood rate of diarrhoea | −0.32 |
| Grosskurth *et al.* (1995) | Community | 6 | HIV rate | 0.94 |
| COMMIT Research Group (1995a) | Community | 11 | Smoking quit rate | 0.21 |

matching correlation is seen to vary widely, from −0.32 to 0.94, including one trial (Haggerty *et al.* 1994) in which matching actually led to a loss in statistical efficiency. It is particularly interesting to note that the trial of Grosskurth *et al.* (1995), which evaluated strategies for preventing HIV infection in regions of Tanzania, generated a matching correlation of 0.94 as computed over only six pairs of communities. The three matching factors used in this trial were location (roadside, lakeshore or island), geographic proximity (less than 50 km apart) and level of prior rates of sexually transmitted disease. Thus the matching strategy was clearly very successful in this study, which reported both a statistically and a clinically significant intervention effect. However, the recently discussed COMMIT trial, with a matching correlation of 0.21 as computed over 11 pairs of communities (Freedman *et al.* 1997), also satisfies the criterion of Martin *et al.* (1993). In this trial, the smoking quit rate over the previous five years was used as a key matching factor.

Unfortunately variables likely to affect outcomes at the cluster level are frequently unknown at the outset of the trial or, if known, may be difficult to match for. For example, as stated by one group of community trial investigators in discussing the challenges faced in their study (Feldman *et al.* 1998), it was 'difficult to specify matching criteria that were both practical to implement, such as those based on demographic data, and plausible'. Moreover, as noted by LaPrelle *et al.* (1992), matching on variables poorly related to outcome will 'do little but reduce power by shifting the unit of analysis from the individual community to the pair of communities'.

These results suggest that the matched-pair design should be considered with caution if the number of pairs available to be matched is small. However, there are also some less recognized limitations to this design that may arise in trials of any size. These limitations arise partly from the difficulty in estimating the intracluster correlation coefficient $\rho$ from matched-pair data. Some consequences of this difficulty include the following:

- Information on $\rho$ useful for the planning of future trials in the same application area will not be routinely available. As will be further discussed in Ch. 5, lack of prior information concerning the value of this parameter can hamper the ability of investigators to properly plan the size of a new trial in the same subject matter area.

- Modelling the effect of individual-level covariates on outcome using regression analysis will require special assumptions.

Neither of these consequences occurs for data arising from either the completely randomized or the stratified design. This is because the latter two designs allow replication at the cluster level for at least some combinations of intervention and stratum. For the matched-pair design, characterized by the assignment of exactly one cluster to each combination of intervention and stratum, there is no such replication. As a result, the inherent variation in response between clusters in a matched pair is totally confounded with the effect of intervention. Thus it is impossible to obtain a valid estimate of $\rho$ except under the null hypothesis of no intervention effect or, as will be discussed below, without making other special assumptions.

We now explore the second of these consequences in more detail. Investigators may be interested in the joint effects of intervention and of individual-level prognostic factors, such as a subject's age, gender or medical history on one or more outcome variables, often referred to as a 'risk factor analysis'. It is natural in such investigations to consider using one of the multiple regression models that have been developed for the analysis of correlated outcome data (see Chs 6–8). The variances of observed regression coefficients for these models may be derived as a function of the intracluster correlation coefficient $\rho$, as described by Scott and Holt (1982) and Neuhaus and Segal (1993). However a valid estimate of $\rho$ is generally not available given the confounding of the intervention effect with the between-cluster component of variance. Thus appropriate standard errors for the estimated regression coefficients cannot be computed, precluding the corresponding test of statistical significance and the construction of confidence intervals. Similar difficulties are associated with other procedures for constructing inferences about regression coefficients, such as robust variance estimation. Klar and Donner (1997) provide further discussion of this issue.

Valid estimates of variances of observed regression coefficients may be developed if they are constructed using between-stratum information, as done in the analyses for the Working Well Trial (Sorensen *et al.* 1996), and as also suggested by Thompson *et al.* (1997b). However, in this case the validity of the resulting inferences requires a large number of matched pairs, rather than a large number of clusters. This requirement was satisfied in the case of the Working Well Trial, which was based on data from 54 pairs of worksites. However, most matched-pair trials tend to be much smaller in size. Moreover, variance estimators obtained using between-stratum information are only valid under the assumption of no stratum by intervention interaction which, as we shall demonstrate, cannot be tested under a matched-pair design.

It is important to note, notwithstanding these difficulties, that if the aim of the analysis is limited to the adjustment or control of individual-level covariates in assessing the effect of intervention, appropriate methods are readily available. These methods take the form of two-stage procedures based on standardizing the data with respect to individual-level covariates in advance of the primary analysis. For example, Gail *et al.* (1992) describe the approach used to adjust for individual-level covariates in the analysis of paired data arising from the COMMIT trial. The first step was to fit a 'null' logistic regression model to the combined study data in order to predict the outcome for each individual. The resulting model contained both cluster-level and individual-level covariates, but no covariates involving the intervention effect. The predicted outcome rate for each cluster was computed by summing the predicted values from the model over all individuals in that cluster. The difference between this predicted rate and the observed outcome rate for the cluster was then treated as a residual free from the effects of those individual-level covariates. The null hypothesis of no intervention effect was then tested by applying a non-parametric permutation test to the difference between the residuals corresponding to the clusters in a matched pair. Further examples of this and related adjusted analyses are given by Brookmeyer and Chen (1998), Smith and Morrow (1991) and Zucker *et al.* (1995).

A third consequence of the inability to estimate $\rho$ is that a test of homogeneity in the effect of intervention across the matched pairs cannot be directly constructed. The assumption of a common intervention effect across strata is required, for example, when constructing confidence intervals about an assumed common odds ratio, and for assessing the power of standard tests of significance. This difficulty is made obvious by considering the standard procedure for testing the homogeneity of odds ratios (e.g. Rosner 1995, pp. 411–413). Let $L_j$ denote the logarithm of the observed odds ratio, $\hat{\Psi}_j$, as computed from the $j$th stratum. Then the appropriate $k-1$ degrees of freedom chi-squared statistic is given by

$$\chi^2_{k-1} = \sum_{j=1}^{k} W_j(L_j - \bar{L})^2$$

where

$$\bar{L} = \sum_{j=1}^{k} W_j L_j \Big/ \sum_{j=1}^{k} W_j$$

and $W_j = (\text{estimated variance of } L_j)^{-1}$. Multiplication of the weights $W_j$ by the appropriate variance inflation factor allows adjustment for the effect of clustering. This, however, requires estimation of the parameter $\rho$.

The special cases in which $\rho$ can be estimated from a matched-pair cluster randomization design are those which allow sufficient replication to permit estimation of between-cluster variability:

- If the intervention is assumed to be ineffective, then the between-cluster variability can be estimated from the clusters within each matched pair, with a pooled estimate of $\rho$ then computed across matched pairs.
- If matching is assumed to be ineffective, i.e. the correlation parameter $\rho_M$ is assumed to be zero, then the between-cluster variability can be estimated from among the clusters within each intervention group, with a pooled estimate of $\rho$ then computed across the two groups.
- If the true effect of intervention is fairly stable over the strata, i.e. the treatment by stratum interaction is negligible, then $\rho$ can be estimated using between-stratum information. In terms of practical application, this approach is most suited to trials involving a reasonably large number of clusters, say $\geqslant 25$, as is typically the case for studies of pair-matched families (Donner and Hauck 1988).

The difficulty in estimating $\rho$ from a matched-pair design suggests that if matching on a given factor is regarded as ineffective, collapsing on that factor might lend more flexibility to the analysis. Although it is intuitively reasonable, more research is needed on the formal statistical properties of this strategy. However, some related results have been reported by Diehr *et al.* (1995b), who used computer simulation to evaluate the most appropriate approach to the statistical analysis of a matched-pair design. Their results show that a cluster-level unmatched analysis is not only valid when applied to a matched-pair design, but can actually lead to an increase in power as compared with a matched analysis when the number of pairs is less than 10. Theoretical support for this interesting finding, which can be attributed in part to the unpaired analysis having twice as many degrees of freedom, was subsequently provided by Proschan (1996). Although these investigations focused on a comparison of the unpaired *t*-test with the paired *t*-test, Diehr *et al.* (1995b) also conjectured that their results would apply to a comparison of matched versus unmatched analyses using permutation tests.

The stratified design has been used much less frequently than either the matched-pair or completely randomized design. However, for many studies it would seem to represent a sensible compromise between these two designs in that it provides at least some baseline control on factors thought to be related to outcome, while easing the practical difficulties of finding appropriate pair-matches and avoiding the unique analytic challenges of the matched-pair design. Furthermore, results obtained by Klar and Donner (1997) suggest that stratified designs may often provide gains in power comparable to matched-pair designs.

A final disadvantage of the matched-pair design is that the loss to follow-up of a single cluster in a pair implies that both clusters in that pair must effectively be discarded from the trial, at least with respect to testing the effect of intervention. This problem, which occurred for example in the cardiovascular disease prevention trial reported by the Family Heart Study Group (1994b), clearly does not arise if there is some replication of clusters within each combination of intervention and stratum.

## 3.7 The importance of cluster-level replication

Some investigators have designed community intervention trials in which exactly one cluster has been assigned to the experimental group and one to the control group, either with or without the benefit of randomization (e.g. Blum and Feachem 1983, Murray *et al.* 1993, Zapka *et al.* 1993, Carleton *et al.* 1995, Mudde *et al.* 1995, Vartianinen *et al.* 1995, Kegeles *et al.* 1996). Such trials invariably result in interpretational difficulties caused by the total confounding of two sources of variation: (i) the variation in response due to the effect of intervention, and (ii) the natural variation that exists between the two communities (clusters) even in the absence of an intervention effect. As pointed out by Kirkwood and Morrow (1989), this design 'is analogous to conducting a clinical trial with just two patients, one receiving the drug and the other placebo'. Measuring and then adjusting for differences in relevant baseline characteristics can help in reducing the effect of such confounding, but is only a partial solution at best to the inherent problem caused by the lack of cluster-level replication. Analysis of such trials is only possible at the level of the individual, and then only if one assumes there is no clustering of individual responses within communities, an assumption which will almost always be untenable.

Interpretational difficulties are not limited to trials including one experimental group and one control group. For example, Worden *et al.* (1990) provide results from a trial in which four Vermont communities were randomly assigned to one of two different breast self-examination intervention groups: to a control group with full measurement or to a low-measurement control group. The natural variability between communities again confounds assessment of the effect of intervention, as well as the assessment of differences across control groups.

The absence of replication, while not exclusive to community intervention trials, is most commonly seen in trials which enrol clusters of relatively large size (e.g. Gray-Donald *et al.* 1985, Jason *et al.* 1990). Unfortunately, the large number of study subjects in such trials may mislead some investigators into believing that valid inferences can be constructed.

More attention to the effects of clustering when determining the trial sample size might also help to eliminate designs which lack replication. Even so, investigators will still need to consider whether or not statistical inferences concerning the effect of intervention will be interpretable if only two, or a few, replicate clusters are allocated to each intervention group. A detailed discussion of sample size considerations is given in Chapter 5.

## 3.8 Strategies for conducting successful trials

There are several additional issues which investigators need to consider when planning a cluster randomization trial. These are related to methods for developing and piloting the interventions, deciding which methods of evaluation will be adopted, and dealing with problems that may arise in writing the trial protocol. The resulting tasks, which must be addressed in any large-scale comparative trial, have been covered extensively elsewhere (e.g. Friedman *et al.* 1996, pp. 10–11, Murray 1998, pp. 50–63). We therefore focus here on problems related to recruitment, loss to follow-up and missing data.

If larger units such as schools, worksites or cities are to be randomized, it is useful to begin with a census of eligible clusters (e.g. Thompson *et al.* 1997a). This will help to determine whether or not there are enough clusters to achieve the desired power as well as to establish the generalizability of the study results. Key decision-makers for each cluster need to be identified and then approached to determine their level of interest in participating in the trial. For example, in school-based studies it is usually necessary to seek the participation of decision-makers at both the district and the school level as well as to obtain the cooperation of teachers, parents and students (Harrington *et al.* 1997).

Thompson *et al.* (1997a), as part of a worksite intervention trial, required eligible worksites to meet several conditions prior to being randomized. These included providing a letter of agreement signed by worksite representatives indicating their willingness to be randomized, as well as an agreement to provide information necessary to conduct the study, including a sampling frame for the workforce and associated summary statistics. In order to be eligible for randomization, worksites also were required to provide a 70 per cent response rate to the baseline survey.

An attractive operational strategy for enhancing compliance is to allocate the units of randomization at a meeting attended by representatives from each cluster. This allows the investigators to demonstrate that any immediate benefits obtained by being assigned to the experimental group are distributed fairly, a strategy followed successfully in the COMMIT trial (Gail *et al.* 1992). The integrity of the randomization was further protected in this trial by the use of a double randomization scheme in which one community in each of the 11 pairs was assigned using computer-generated random numbers to one of the colours red or black. After placing this information in sealed envelopes, a roulette wheel was spun once for each matched pair of communities in order to determine whether red or black denoted the experimental community.

The intervention should be initiated as soon as possible after randomization. This ensures that baseline assessments accurately describe clusters immediately prior to their receiving the intervention. It also protects against a possible decline in interest and consequent risk of loss to follow-up if there is too lengthy a delay before start-up. However, when random assignment of all clusters is conducted simultaneously, as was the case for COMMIT, the demands on data collection and data management resources can be considerable. Attention to data management issues should therefore begin in the design stage of the trial.

A plan for monitoring the randomized clusters should be considered in order to assess the ongoing quality of the data and to identify any difficulties in following the protocol. Ellickson (1994), in the context of a school-based trial, suggested that site coordinators be hired who would be responsible for monitoring progress, addressing concerns expressed by teachers regarding the implementation of the intervention, and attending to concerns expressed by parents.

Issues involved in data management have been discussed by Pradhan *et al.* (1994) in the context of a community intervention trial in Nepal, and by Pinol *et al.* (1998) in the context of a multinational antenatal care trial (further discussed in Section 5.4). A more general review of data management issues for clinical trials is provided by McFadden (1997).

# 4

# The role of informed consent and other ethical issues

Every randomized trial requires assurance that the proposed study design meets commonly accepted ethical standards. This task is complicated by the fact that almost all ethical guidelines for randomized trials have been written with individually randomized trials in mind and are, consequently, only partially applicable to trials which randomize intact units of subjects. Only recently has much attention been given to the ethical challenges posed by cluster randomization (e.g. Glanz *et al.* 1996, Edwards *et al.* 1999).

We follow the basic premise that trials which are methodologically unsound are by definition unethical. Trials which ignore the effects of clustering both during the study design and at the data analysis stage tend to be underpowered (i.e. have a type II error greater than nominal) and yet are also biased in favour of declaring inactive interventions as being helpful (i.e. have a type I error greater than nominal). The methods needed to account for these problems are described elsewhere in the text and are not further discussed in this chapter. Similarly we omit discussion here of possible ethical motivations that may account for the original decision to adopt cluster randomization.

Piantadosi (1997, Ch. 3) discussed ethical issues in clinical trials from a very broad perspective, while we focus here on those issues which are particularly relevant to cluster randomization trials. We first focus attention on the importance of avoiding harm, ensuring equity among subjects and respecting a subject's right to be fully informed about his or her involvement in a research project. In Section 4.1 we therefore consider the relative potential for harm and benefit to subjects participating in either individually randomized or cluster randomized trials. One conclusion we draw is that the risk of harm may prove greater than is apparent at first glance. The importance of obtaining informed consent whenever possible and the absolute minimum requirement of obtaining the full participation of group representatives are described in Section 4.2, while issues involving subject blindness and informed consent are dealt with in Section 4.3. In Section 4.4 we review randomized consent designs, discuss some similarities they share with cluster randomized trials and also review several novel applications of the single consent design. We conclude by discussing ethical issues related to trial monitoring in Section 4.5.

## 4.1 The risk of harm

The challenge of designing an ethical randomized trial requires balancing the potential benefits and risk of harm faced by individual participants with the potential long-term benefit to those subjects and to society at large. Too often the potential risks of participating in health education or disease prevention trials have been essentially neglected (Gillon 1990, Skrabanek 1990). This is unfortunate because not all such trials meet the criteria of minimal risk. According to the US Federal Government (Office for Protection from Research Risks 1994)

> Minimal risk means that the probability and magnitude of harm or discomfort anticipated in the research are not greater than those ordinarily encountered in daily life or during the performance of routine physical or psychological examinations or tests.

Furthermore, as the benefits from participation in a trial decrease, so must the risk of harm.

Consider, for example, randomized trials of disease screening programmes. Cluster randomization designs have been advocated here on the grounds that they more closely replicate the circumstances under which a successful programme will be ultimately implemented (Miller 1996). Thus examples of studies designed to evaluate the success of disease screening include cluster randomization trials focusing on cardiovascular disease (e.g. Bass *et al.* 1986, the Family Heart Study Group 1994a, b), parasitic infections (Gyorkos *et al.* 1989) and breast cancer (see Nystrom *et al.* 1993).

The benefit from screening will only be achieved by identifying subjects whose illness can be cured if detected and whose illness would have progressed if left untreated. Participation in screening programmes thus offers healthy individuals few benefits and some risks. One avenue for harm is the labelling or mislabelling of otherwise healthy individuals as having a disease (e.g. Bergman and Stamm 1967, Macdonald *et al.* 1984, Stewart-Brown and Farmer 1997). Ethical issues peculiar to disease screening are further explored by Marshall (1996) and Shickle and Chadwick (1994).

Even seemingly innocuous disease prevention programmes cannot, *a priori*, be considered as having minimal risk. According to the theory of risk homeostasis proposed by Wilde (1994), which is admittedly controversial, there is a tendency for people to accept certain fixed amounts of risk. For example, laws requiring the use of childproof caps may result in increases in accidental childhood poisoning because less attention is given to safe storage of medication. Similarly, legislation mandating the use of seat belts has been suggested to be a cause of riskier driving, resulting in increased injuries. Although evidence for Wilde's theory is not strong (see, e.g. Shannon and Szatmari 1994), investigators would be remiss if they did not at least consider the possible risks of their proposed interventions.

In some instances, participants in cluster randomized trials may face more direct risks. Avorn *et al.* (1992), for example, describe the results of a health education trial aimed at physicians, nurses and aides in nursing homes and designed to reduce the use of psychoactive drugs by residents. Six pair-matched nursing homes were included in the trial with one member of each matched pair being randomly assigned to the educational programme. In addition to the ethical challenges of studying elderly subjects, not all of whom may be fully competent, the investigators were forced to contend with the possibility that attempts at lowering the overuse of psychoactive drugs might leave some individuals without medically required treatment (Avorn 1992).

Similar risks of a direct nature arise in many cluster randomized trials. Such risks may have been faced, for example, by participants in cluster randomized trials of vitamin A supplementation on childhood mortality (e.g. Fawzi *et al.* 1993), by patients in a community intervention trial of cancer pain management (Elliot *et al.* 1997), and by subjects in the Tanzanian community intervention trial of sexually transmitted diseases on HIV infection (Grosskurth *et al.* 1995). No claim is made here that these interventions are harmful. To the contrary, there is increasing evidence as to the beneficial effects of vitamin A in preventing childhood mortality. It is a sad irony, however, that these benefits may not be shared by beta-carotene, a precursor to vitamin A. Individually randomized chemopreventive trials have found that dietary supplements of beta-carotene increase rather than decrease the risk of lung cancer (Mayne *et al.* 1996)!

Concern for the risk/benefit ratio also extends to control group subjects, e.g. when these participants receive placebos when in fact active agents are available (e.g. Rothman 1996). In some cluster randomization trials, investigators have attempted to ensure that subjects in control groups can still benefit from participation by randomly assigning them to either early or delayed intervention, as in the screening and treatment trial reported by Gyorkos *et al.* (1989), or, alternatively, by allowing them to receive at least a minimal level of intervention (Glanz *et al.* 1996).

Investigators should be encouraged to recognize that participation in a cluster randomization trial may entail considerable effort at both the individual and the cluster levels. At a minimum, it is important to communicate study findings both to trial participants and to decision-makers (CIOMS 1991, Section 13). Investigators should also be sensitive to the consequences of a successful intervention so that the benefits enjoyed by study participants do not necessarily end when the trial is completed.

## 4.2 Informed consent

International declarations such as the World Medical Association Declaration of Helsinki were devised specifically to guide physicians conducting therapeutic trials (World Medical Association 1997). These declarations require that consent be obtained from each patient prior to random assignment. Section 1.9 of the 1996 version of the Helsinki Declaration states that:

> In any research on human beings, each potential subject must be adequately informed of the aims, methods, anticipated benefits and potential hazards of the study and the discomfort it may entail. He or she should be informed that he or she is at liberty to abstain from participation in the study and he or she is free to withdraw his or her consent to participation at any time. The physician should then obtain the subject's freely-given informed consent, preferably in writing.

By strict analogy to the current ethical requirements for clinical trials, it would therefore be unethical not to obtain informed consent from every cluster member prior to

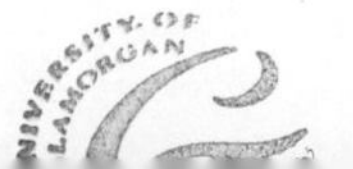

random assignment. However, as pointed out by Buck and Donner (1982), these requirements have emanated over time from an implicit contractual relationship between patient and physician based on the patient's individual treatment programme. The question therefore arises as to whether such a strict analogy is required or, in fact, is possible for cluster randomization trials, since difficulties in obtaining informed consent in large clusters such as schools, doctors practices or communities are well recognized. It may be permissible in some studies that the decision regarding random assignment and implementation of an intervention comes from community leaders or decision-makers (e.g. school principal, clinic director, mayor). However, individual study subjects must still be at liberty to withhold their participation, although even then they may not be able to completely avoid the inherent risks of an intervention that is applied on a cluster-wide level. Thus the Council for International Organizations of Medical Sciences (Howard-Jones 1982) makes the following recommendations (Sections 16 and 17):

> Where research is undertaken on a community basis – for example by experimental treatment of water supplies, by health services research or by large-scale trials of new insecticides, of new prophylactic or immunizing agents, and of nutritional adjuvants or substitutes – individual consent on a person-to-person basis may not be feasible and the ultimate decision to undertake the research will rest with the responsible public health authority.
>
> Nevertheless, all possible means should be used to inform the community concerned of the aims of the research, the advantages expected from it and any possible hazards or inconveniences. If feasible, dissenting individuals should have the option of withholding their participation. Whatever the circumstances, the ethical considerations and safeguards applied to research on individuals must be translated, in every possible respect, into the community context.

This form of community agreement was further explored by Last (1991), Glanz *et al.* (1996) and as part of the proposed International Guidelines for Ethical Review of Epidemiological Studies (CIOMS 1991). Note that this alternative to individual informed consent is not universally accepted, especially when deemed to be used in the developing world only to avoid ethical requirements which would otherwise be imposed (e.g. Lurie *et al.* 1994).

The identification of individuals mandated to provide agreement for random assignment may not be an easy task. Permission can be sought from local ethical review committees (i.e. Institutional Review Boards or IRBs) when hospitals are the unit of randomization. The premise here is that IRBs have the expertise to properly evaluate the trial, as well as the authority to speak for their institution. What of trials in which the units of randomization consist of schools, worksites, churches or communities? Typically, it is elected or appointed officials who make such decisions. However, Strasser *et al.* (1987) point out that it is by no means certain when, or even if, the agreement of these officials is sufficient. Investigators are therefore encouraged to consider supplementing the consent of decision-makers by seeking input from individuals who might be directly affected by the trial. Thus it is clear that two distinct levels of informed consent must often be distinguished in practice: informed consent for randomization (possibly provided by a single 'decision-maker'), and informed consent for participants given that randomization has occurred.

It is interesting to note the detailed attention given to informed consent in a trial of vitamin A supplementation in Northern Ghana (Ghana VAST Study Team 1993).

This trial involved over 20 000 children aged 6–90 months in 185 geographical clusters; 92 clusters were randomly assigned to vitamin A, while 93 received placebo treatment. The trial was explained in detail to all relevant authorities, who gave their formal approval. However, efforts were also made to

> keep the communities informed of the study's purpose, and any new developments, through meetings open to all community members and by announcements at market places. The trial was also explained and consent was sought from the head of each compound and the parents or guardians of each eligible child before enrolment.

It is clear that in this trial the investigators attempted as much as possible to obtain the views of those most directly affected by the intervention. This is consistent with Section 6 of the CIOMS (1991) guidelines, which state:

> When people are appointed by agencies outside a group, such as a department of government, to speak for members of the group, investigators and ethical review committees should consider how authentically these people speak for the group, and if necessary seek also the agreement of other representatives. Representatives of a community or group may sometimes be in a position to participate in designing the study and in its ethical assessment.

These guidelines would seem to imply that in worksite intervention trials, for example, representatives from both management and labour should be actively involved in the trial design (Sorensen *et al.* 1995). As an added benefit, the active participation and enthusiasm of all relevant stakeholders may also help to increase compliance.

School-based trials raise special issues, e.g. as to whether parental consent is required. If the intervention consists of a new teaching method, it has been argued by Schlegel (1977) that such consent is not required 'since teachers have the professional prerogative to decide on the actual content and teaching methods'. Certainly this, possibly dated, sentiment is not universally accepted. For example, parental consent was required in a trial evaluating a violence prevention curriculum among children in elementary school (Grossman *et al.* 1997) and in a trial comparing treatments for the elimination of head lice in children (Chosidow *et al.* 1994). Each of these trials is noteworthy for the direct involvement of the children's parents, either to help in the data collection (Grossman *et al.* 1997) or to help administer the treatment (Chosidow *et al.* 1994). Thus in these studies, informed consent was required in order to ensure compliance.

A more general discussion of consent in school-based trials is provided by Esbensen *et al.* (1996). Distinctions are drawn here between active consent, where students are only invited to enrol in a trial following parental approval, and passive consent, where students are invited to enrol unless parents object. Perhaps not unexpectedly, studies requiring active consent tend to enrol a smaller proportion of students as compared with studies using passive consent. Active consent might still prove preferable in studies requiring the active participation of parents, or where questions posed to the students may be regarded as sensitive.

These practical difficulties of obtaining informed consent prior to random assignment do not necessarily arise when smaller clusters such as households or families are the unit of randomization. For instance, Walker *et al.* (1992) report on the results from a cluster randomized trial designed to reduce cardiovascular disease risk factors among teenage children of patients with ischaemic heart disease. Families were randomly assigned to either an 'early' or a 'late' advice group, with all study participants providing informed consent. Close attention to the issue of informed consent can also be noted in a trial reported by Payment *et al.* (1991). These investigators evaluated the risk of gastrointestinal disease in households randomly assigned to receive domestic water filters as compared with households using tap water. One of the eligibility criteria was 'willingness to participate in a longitudinal trial in which a random half of the households would have a filter installed'.

The decision to omit informed consent when deemed necessary merits careful consideration. Certainly this decision has proved to be controversial in trials randomizing families. Dennis *et al.* (1997), for example, report on a trial designed to examine the effect of contact with a stroke family care worker on the physical, social and psychological status of stroke patients and their care-givers. The investigators, with the support of a local ethics committee, decided that the risk of harm was too slight to warrant informed consent. Furthermore, the investigators were concerned that subjects' responses could be biased if they were fully informed of the purpose and design of the study (Dennis 1997). Although acknowledging the difficulties faced by Dennis *et al.* (1997), several critics subsequently argued that respect for the study subjects should have outweighed these methodological concerns (e.g. McLean 1997).

The relative absence of ethical guidelines for cluster randomized trials appears to have created a research environment in which the choice of randomization unit may determine whether or not informed consent is deemed necessary prior to random assignment. This phenomenon can be seen, for example, in the several published trials of vitamin A supplementation on childhood mortality. Informed consent was obtained from mothers prior to assigning children to either vitamin A or placebo in the household randomization trial reported by Herrera *et al.* (1992). This was not the case in the community intervention trial of vitamin A reported by the Ghana VAST Study Team (1993), where consent to participate was obtained only after random assignment. It seems questionable, on both an ethical and a methodological level, whether the unit of randomization should play such a critical role in deciding whether or not informed consent is required, and, if so, to what extent.

## 4.3 Subject blindness and informed consent

In a controlled clinical trial, ideally both subject and investigator are unaware of which intervention is being received by a particular patient (i.e. the trial is 'double blind'). This is often accomplished in oral drug trials, e.g. by ensuring that the products taken both look and taste alike. However, it is usually much more difficult to arrange subject blindness in cluster randomization trials, particularly in the case of lifestyle or other non-therapeutic interventions. For example, in the cardiovascular disease prevention trial reported by Walker *et al.* (1992), all families were made aware of the behavioural intervention programme prior to random assignment. As a consequence, subjects assigned to the late advice group might have adopted behaviours similar to those of subjects randomized to the early advice group. In this case, the estimated effect of intervention might be biased if subjects were treated or assessed differently depending on the group to which they were assigned.

Of course, these difficulties do not characterize all cluster randomization trials. For example, both subject and investigator blindness were achieved in several of the well-known trials of vitamin A supplementation randomizing communities to either an experimental or a placebo control group (e.g. West *et al.* 1991).

One could argue (e.g. Buck and Donner 1982) that if the intervention is of a very general nature, as in the case of health education messages given through the media to a set of experimental communities, there may be little ethical objection to individual subjects being unaware of the programme. If this is the case, then of course the problem of explicitly ensuring subject blindness does not arise. For example, in the hypertension trial discussed in Chapter 1 (Bass *et al.* 1986), the patients in the experimental and control practices were not aware of the specific nature of the investigation, although they knew their physician was participating in a research study. Of course, the ethical implications of subjects being unaware of the details of an investigation or being unaware that they are even in a randomized trial must be considered separately for each study.

## 4.4 Randomized consent designs

In most therapeutic trials, informed consent is typically obtained immediately prior to random assignment. As part of the informed consent process, the physician must admit ignorance regarding the optimal therapy and patients must agree to allow chance to dictate which treatment they will receive. The strain that these requirements of informed consent may place on the relationship between physician and patient is, at times, a barrier to patient accrual (Schain 1994, Ellenberg 1997). Randomized consent designs were introduced and later refined by Zelen (1979, 1990) to help lower this barrier and thus hasten trial completion.

Two randomized consent designs have been described in the literature, known as the double-consent design and the single-consent design. In the double-consent design, patients are randomly assigned to an experimental or a standard therapy prior to asking for consent. Patients are then asked if they consent to receive the intervention to which they have been assigned. If they refuse, they may be offered the alternative therapy under consideration. In the single-consent design, patients are also randomly assigned either to standard or to an experimental therapy. However, consent is sought only from patients randomly assigned to the experimental therapy. These patients have the option of declining their assigned intervention in favour of the standard therapy. All analyses are conducted according to the 'intent to treat' strategy, i.e. are based on the original intervention assignment. Any loss in efficiency resulting from patients preferring an alternative treatment arm is expected to be offset by the potential gain in accrual.

The randomized consent design has proved quite controversial since first being proposed and has only been adopted in a small number of therapeutic trials (Altman *et al.* 1995). Reluctance to use randomized consent arises, at least in part, because of concern for the ethical implications of randomizing subjects prior to obtaining their consent. However, this strategy is typical of most cluster randomized trials, particularly those involving large clusters such as entire communities. Moreover, all individuals residing in such communities are potentially placed at risk, further complicating the decision to adopt this design.

In spite of these difficulties, studies have been conducted which have made use of the single-consent design. For example, Villar *et al.* (1998) and Donner (1998) discuss the design of a stratified cluster randomized trial comparing the impact of two antenatal care programmes. One programme consists of the 'best standard treatment' while the other programme uses only those tests, clinical activities and follow-up actions scientifically demonstrated to be effective in improving maternal and newborn outcomes. The medical chiefs or directors from all participating clinics allowed their clinic to be randomly assigned to one of the two trial arms, with informed consent obtained only from women attending clinics randomized to the experimental group. Since women attending clinics assigned to the 'best standard treatment' were assigned the same care which they would have received outside the trial, no consent was deemed necessary in these clinics.

Two cancer screening trials discussed by Torgerson and Roland (1998) also employed the single-consent design. The first of these two trials was conducted in the vicinity of Nottingham in the United Kingdom (Hardcastle *et al.* 1996). Subjects were randomized by household to faecal occult blood screening for colorectal cancer or to a control group. The second trial, reported by Kronborg *et al.* (1996), was conducted in Funen, Denmark, and also considered the effect of faecal occult blood screening on the risk of colorectal cancer. Husbands and wives were randomly assigned as a couple in the Danish trial, with all other random assignments made at the individual level. Control subjects in both trials continued to receive their usual care and were not told about the existence of the study. This omission was considered ethical and necessary in order to prevent control group subjects from changing their behaviour.

Zelen (1982) suggested that randomized consent designs would eventually be widely used in clinical trials. To the extent that most cluster randomized trials must make use of some form of randomization prior to consent, it would appear that he was correct.

## 4.5 Ethical issues and trial monitoring

During the course of a trial, it is common practice for an independent committee of experts (the Data and Safety Monitoring Committee) to safeguard the interests of participants, as is the case in most large-scale clinical trials. The broad issues involved in trial monitoring and interim reporting, as discussed by many authors (e.g. Friedman *et al.* 1996, Ch. 15, Piantadosi 1997, Section 10.8), also apply generally to cluster randomized trials. Efficacy monitoring in accordance with a predetermined plan, however, does not seem to be a common feature of most cluster randomization trials. This is at least partly because the theoretical underpinnings of standard data-dependent stopping plans, such as that developed by O'Brien and Fleming (1979), invariably assume individual randomization, while methods applicable to cluster randomization trials have yet to be widely adopted (Wei *et al.* 1990, Gange and DeMets 1996). It may also be that the ethical need to terminate a trial due to unexpected early benefits or harm is often perceived as fairly remote. A notable exception is the Ghana VAST trial which examined the effect of vitamin A supplementation on childhood mortality (Ghana VAST Study Team 1993). An interim analysis was conducted by an independent monitoring committee after 12 months of follow-up. The committee recommended that the trial continue to the end of the planned 24 months of follow-up.

Aside from issues of safety and efficacy, interim analyses are also beneficial because they may allow investigators to monitor accrual on both a cluster and an individual level, as well as intermittently to assess baseline comparability. Interim analyses also allow the opportunity to reassess the adequacy of the trial size on the basis of early information, and, if necessary, to revise the protocol accordingly.

# 5

# Sample size estimation for cluster randomization designs

A quantitatively justified sample size calculation is almost universally regarded as a fundamental design feature of a properly controlled clinical trial. As stated by Friedman *et al.* (1996) 'clinical trials should have sufficient statistical power to detect differences between groups considered to be of clinical interest. Therefore calculation of sample size with provision for adequate levels of significance and power is an essential part of planning'. This statement would seem to apply with equal force to trials which randomize intact clusters as it does to trials which randomize individuals. It is particularly relevant to the design of community intervention trials, where many subjects and large expenditures of time and money have frequently been the norm. Yet, as discussed in Chapter 1, methodological reviews of cluster randomization trials have consistently shown that only a small proportion of these studies have adopted a predetermined sample size based on formal considerations of statistical power. It is interesting to speculate as to why this should be so. One obvious reason is that the appropriate formulas tend to be relatively inaccessible, not being given, for example, in most standard texts and articles on clinical trial methodology. A second reason is that the proper use of these formulas requires some prior assessment of the intracluster correlation coefficient $\rho$, either directly or through comparable information on the value of $\sigma_A^2$, the between-cluster component of variation. Neither of these parameters may be very familiar to investigators, complicating the task of obtaining relevant past data that may be used for sample size planning. This point was alluded to by Gail *et al.* (1992), in their discussion of the statistical aspects of the COMMIT trial, where they stated that 'the major problem in designing community intervention trials such as COMMIT is obtaining reliable estimates of the between-community component of variation'. A third reason why the issue of sample size estimation may tend to be ignored in cluster randomization trials is that studies enrolling hundreds or even thousands of patients may give the misleading impression of extensive statistical power, when in fact the effective sample size, after taking into account the clustering effect, is actually quite small.

Adding to the difficulties of ensuring that cluster randomization trials are of adequate size are several practical factors that more or less uniquely apply to the successful conduct of such studies. As will be seen, the power of a cluster randomization trial depends more on the number of units randomized than on their size. However, the number of units that can be realistically studied may be small, due to reasons of logistics and cost. Limited resources may also lead to a diluted intensity of effect in the experimental group, especially if these resources must be spread over a wide geographic area. These problems may be compounded by the difficulties of arranging subject blindness, thus allowing control group members to become aware of, or even assume, activities of the experimental group, further diluting the effect of intervention through a 'spill-over' effect. Finally there may be an increased risk of loss to follow-up due to unique features of this design.

Many cluster randomization trials take the form of prevention studies, further adding to the difficulties. Prevention trials usually enrol subjects from healthy populations, with the consequence that the event rates one wishes to reduce are relatively low in the first instance, with the benefits of intervention not readily apparent. Compliance with the intervention may also be difficult to maintain in such populations, especially over a relatively long period of time. More generally, there may be a greater than usual risk in such studies that the individuals evaluated for outcomes are not necessarily those exposed to the intervention.

Published editorial comments have explicitly dealt with these concerns in the context of community-based intervention trials. Susser (1995), commenting on large-scale trials involving public health interventions, noted that 'generally, the size of effects has been meagre in relation to the effort expended' and 'we often do not even have the resources to detect medium effects'. Fishbein (1996), making a similar point, goes on to emphasize that

> outcome measures must be sensitive to the purpose of the intervention, and when a small-sized effect is meaningful (and all we can expect) for a given outcome measure, we must make sure that we have the sample size necessary to detect such an effect.

These comments emphasize that the need to provide a formal estimate of statistical power is as important in trials randomizing clusters as it is in trials randomizing individuals.

In Section 5.1 we review some general issues involved in the estimation of sample size for cluster randomization trials. Methods applicable to the three most frequently adopted designs (i.e. completely randomized, matched-pair and stratified) are then described in Sections 5.2, 5.3 and 5.4 respectively. Issues involving loss to follow-up of study subjects and/or clusters are discussed in Section 5.5, while Section 5.6 provides some strategies which may help to overcome common barriers to achieving desired levels of statistical power.

## 5.1 General issues of sample size estimation

There are a number of issues common to sample size estimation that apply to any randomized trial. These include: (1) identification of the primary study outcome, (2) determination of a minimally important effect of intervention, and (3) specification of a statistical test or confidence interval method along with its directionality (i.e. one- or two-sided). In this section we focus on two related issues that have unique significance in cluster randomization trials: the determination of cluster size and the prior assessment of $\rho$.

As noted in Section 3.2, cluster size is to some degree, determined by the selected interventions. For example, households were the natural unit of randomization in the study reported by Payment *et al.* (1991), which considered the effect of domestic water filters on subjects' risk of gastrointestinal disease. Consequently, the average cluster size at entry in this trial was approximately four. On the other hand, mass education studies such as COMMIT (COMMIT Research Group 1995a) must consider random assignment of entire communities. At times, however, investigators have much greater latitude in selecting the unit of randomization. For example, randomized trials examining the effect of vitamin A on childhood mortality have been designed allocating units as diverse as households, villages and entire districts to intervention groups.

It is important in practice to distinguish between the size of a cluster and the number of subjects sampled per cluster, i.e. subsampled. For instance, many community intervention trials are economically restricted to enrolling only a subset of eligible residents unless the primary outcome is based on routinely collected data (e.g. mortality). Thus in the COMMIT trial, approximately 550 heavy smokers were subsampled per community and then followed up to compare quit rates among subjects in the control and experimental groups.

Contamination between subjects in different intervention groups can be a problem whenever the clusters are geographically proximate. As a precaution against contamination in community intervention trials, Hayes (1998) suggested sampling subjects from the geographic center of each community. However, the degree of intracluster correlation is usually assumed, for the purposes of trial planning, to be unaffected by both the number of individuals subsampled and the method of subsampling used. Given the usual uncertainties associated with sample size estimation, this assumption should be reasonable in practice.

In some studies, the number of subjects sampled from each cluster may be determined so as to minimize the overall costs. This requires having some indication of the cost of enrolling an additional individual from each cluster relative to the cost of recruiting an additional cluster. Appropriate methods may be adapted using techniques developed for cluster sampling (e.g. Levy and Lemeshow 1980, Section 11.5, McKinlay 1994). However, it is usually simpler to determine the number of subjects sampled per cluster as part of a sensitivity analysis. These analyses are conducted by estimating the required trial size under a number of different scenarios. Investigators are often surprised to learn from such analyses that even small changes in the expected effect of intervention, in the number of subjects sampled per cluster or in the intracluster correlation coefficient can have large effects on the required sample size.

It may be argued that sensitivity analyses serve a particularly important role in the planning of cluster randomization trials. This is largely a consequence of the difficulty investigators have in obtaining accurate estimates of either between-cluster variability or intracluster correlation. Together with cluster size, these quantities are used to adjust the sample size for the variance inflation due to clustering (see Sections 5.2–5.4). However, inaccuracies may still remain because estimates of intracluster correlation obtained from studies with only a small number of clusters are very imprecise.

Difficulties in obtaining accurate estimates of intracluster correlation are further complicated by the relatively small number of publications which present these values when reporting trial results. However, intracluster correlation estimates for smoking-related outcomes as obtained from school-based intervention studies have been provided by Siddiqui *et al.* (1996) and Murray and Hannan (1990), while Slymen and Hovell (1997) provide similar outcomes obtained from a cluster randomized trial of 154 orthodontist offices. Estimated intracluster correlation coefficients and design effects for health-related outcomes as obtained from a worksite health promotion study have been provided by Kelder *et al.* (1993), while estimates of design effects for community trials of mortality from cardiovascular disease and cancer are given by Mickey *et al.* (1991) and Mickey and Goodwin (1993). Note that design effects always depend on the combined effect of the intracluster correlation coefficient and sizes of the clusters randomized.

An alternative approach to dealing with random variation in published estimates of intracluster correlation, based on conducting simulation experiments similar in principle to the bootstrap method, is described by Feng and Grizzle (1992). They propose that, instead of using a single value of $\rho$, one should simulate the results of studies of the size that yielded the estimate. One can then substitute the values calculated from each simulation into the appropriate formula to generate a distribution of these sample sizes, e.g. the 90th percentile, that reflects the degree of conservativeness desired. Yet another approach is to set the value of $\rho$ equal to the upper limit of a (say) 95 per cent confidence interval for this parameter as computed from a suitable dataset. One complication is the absence of strong evidence demonstrating that confidence intervals constructed using available variance estimators (e.g. Feng and Grizzle 1992, Murray *et al.* 1994) remain valid when these estimators are derived from studies involving only a few clusters of variable size. A further complication is that confidence interval methods for $\rho$ in the case of a binary outcome variable are not yet well developed. Setting $\rho = 1$ avoids the need to obtain a more accurate advance estimate of this parameter, but is clearly very conservative.

The degree to which responses of cluster members are correlated, and consequently the size of the resulting variance inflation factor, will tend to vary across different units of randomization. Not surprisingly, responses among subjects from smaller clusters (e.g. households) tend to be more highly correlated than responses among subjects from larger clusters (e.g. communities). For example, people from the same household tend to be more alike than randomly selected subjects who live in the same city. Other examples of this inverse relationship between cluster size and the degree of intracluster correlation have been noted repeatedly in both cluster randomization trials and surveys using cluster sampling (e.g. Hansen and Hurwitz 1942, Hansen *et al.* 1953, pp. 306–309, Katz *et al.* 1993b). Although the magnitude of the intracluster correlation coefficient tends to decline with cluster size, it does so at a relatively slow rate. Thus, larger variance inflation factors are usually obtained when randomizing large clusters such as communities than when randomizing much smaller clusters such as households.

Estimates of intracluster correlation may also be obtained from complex surveys which employ cluster sampling. For example, Gulliford *et al.* (1999) have reported a set of such estimates obtained from a cross-sectional survey of English adults which included data on a range of lifestyle risk factors and health outcomes. Verma and Le (1996) present a very extensive list of intracluster correlation coefficients for variables such as fertility, family planning, child health and mortality, as compiled from data generated by 48 nationally representative surveys. Summary information on these data sources is provided in Table 5.1.

**Table 5.1** Selected sources for estimates of intracluster correlation coefficients and design effects (Koepsell 1998)

| Reference | Outcomes | Cluster |
|---|---|---|
| Chen *et al.* (1997) | Cholesterol levels among children | Family |
| Vachon *et al.* (1998) | Dietary intakes among postmenopausal women | Family |
| Katz *et al.* (1993a, b), Katz and Zeger (1994) | Childhood illness | Family, village |
| Siddiqui *et al.* (1996) | Tobacco use among adolescents | Classroom, school |
| Murray and Hannan (1990), Murray *et al.* (1994) | Tobacco and drug use among adolescents | School |
| Slymen and Hovell (1997) | Tobacco and alcohol use among adolescents | Orthodontist offices |
| Kelder *et al.* (1993) | Physical health and tobacco use | Worksites |
| Gulliford *et al.* (1999) | Lifestyle risk factors and health outcomes | Neighbourhood, household |
| Verma and Le (1996) | Fertility rates, family and child health | Neighbourhood |
| Feldman and McKinlay (1994) | Height, weight, body mass index, blood pressure, cholesterol levels | Community |
| Hannan *et al.* (1994) | Behavioural risk factors, knowledge and attitudes concerning heart disease | Community |
| Murray and Short (1995) | Alcohol use among adolescents | Community |
| Murray and Short (1997) | Tobacco use among adolescents | Community |
| Mickey *et al.* (1991), Mickey and Goodwin (1993) | Mortality from cardiovascular disease and cancer | County |

To summarize, there are several reasons for considering a range of possible values of intracluster correlation when estimating sample size. First, estimates of intracluster correlation coefficient are dependent on the study design. Thus an estimate of intracluster correlation obtained from a study employing stratified randomization may be smaller than if a completely randomized design had been used (assuming that the stratification is effective). Second, this estimate may be computed from a study having only a small number of clusters. Third, the number of subjects participating per cluster in the planned trial will often be highly variable, which will further inflate the variance of the estimated effect of intervention. Finally, relatively little information is currently available concerning the generalizability of estimates of intracluster correlation. For example, the study referred to above by Verma and Le (1996) reports substantial variation in the degree of intracluster correlation across the 48 surveys examined.

## 5.2 The completely randomized design

### 5.2.1 Comparison of means

Suppose that $k$ clusters of $m$ individuals are randomly assigned to each of group $i$ ($i = 1, 2$), where $i = 1$ denotes the experimental group and $i = 2$ denotes the control group. We denote the primary response variable for an individual by $Y$, where $Y$ is assumed to be normally distributed with common but unknown variance $\sigma^2$. Since there are two sources of variation that influence the value of this parameter, we may write $\sigma^2 = \sigma_A^2 + \sigma_W^2$, where $\sigma_W^2$ denotes the variance in response within clusters and $\sigma_A^2$ the variance among clusters. We assume that the aim of the investigators is to test the hypothesis $H_0: \mu_1 = \mu_2$ at the two-sided $100\alpha$ per cent level of significance with power $1 - \beta$, where $\mu_1$ and $\mu_2$ are the population means of $Y$ in the experimental and control groups, respectively. Sample estimates of $\mu_1$ and $\mu_2$ are given by $\overline{Y}_1$ and $\overline{Y}_2$, respectively, where these estimates are computed over all individuals in each group.

Let $Z_{\alpha/2}$ denote the two-sided critical value of the standard normal distribution corresponding to the error rate $\alpha$, and $Z_\beta$ denote the critical value corresponding to $\beta$. Then, if $\overline{Y}_1 - \overline{Y}_2$ can be regarded as approximately normally distributed, the number of subjects required per intervention group is given (Donner *et al.* 1981) by

$$n = \frac{(Z_{\alpha/2} + Z_\beta)^2(2\sigma^2)[1 + (m-1)\rho]}{(\mu_1 - \mu_2)^2} \tag{5.1}$$

where $\rho = \sigma_A^2/(\sigma_A^2 + \sigma_W^2)$ is the intracluster correlation coefficient, and $\mu_1 - \mu_2$ denotes the magnitude of the difference to be detected (for one-sided calculations, $Z_{\alpha/2}$ is replaced by $Z_\alpha$). With this allocation, the 'effective sample size' for each group would be given by $n/[1 + (m-1)\rho]$. Thus at $\rho = 0$, equation (5.1) reduces to the usual sample size specification (e.g. Armitage and Berry 1994, Section 6.6). Equivalent to equation (5.1), the number of clusters required per group is given by

$$k = \frac{(Z_{\alpha/2} + Z_\beta)^2(2\sigma^2)[1 + (m-1)\rho]}{m(\mu_1 - \mu_2)^2} \tag{5.2}$$

The parameter $\mu_1 - \mu_2$ would usually be specified in advance as the minimum value of the intervention effect regarded as substantively important to detect. In practice, the investigators must assess this value on the basis of judgment, augmented by the best available data. Zucker *et al.* (1995) describe how this was done for the CATCH trial, where the investigators were required to specify the detectable mean difference for total serum cholesterol.

The use of the critical values $Z_{\alpha/2}, Z_\beta$ in the formulas above rather than critical values $t_{\alpha/2}$, $t_\beta$ corresponding to the $t$-distribution will underestimate the required sample size unless the degrees of freedom are large. A simple adjustment for this undercorrection (Snedecor and Cochran 1989, p. 104) is to add one cluster per intervention group when the sample size is determined using a 5 per cent type I error rate, and two clusters per group assuming a 1 per cent type I error rate. No correction for the degrees of freedom is necessary if the total number of clusters is approximately 30 or more (Lachin 1981).

A more exact iterative procedure may also be used, as described by Murray and Hannan (1990). Iteration is required to implement this procedure since the degrees of freedom, given by $2(k-1)$, are a function of sample size. However, these difficulties can be avoided using the SAS program provided by Donner and Klar (1996) to determine exact power.

In the case of unequal cluster sizes, we may replace $m$ in equation (5.1) by an advance estimate of the average cluster size $\overline{m}$. This approximation will tend to slightly underestimate the actual required sample size, but the underestimation will be negligible provided the variation in cluster size is not substantial. A conservative approach would be to replace $m$ by $m_{max}$, the largest anticipated cluster size in the sample. Taking a conservative approach would also provide some protection of statistical power in the event that the loss to follow-up rate for the trial is underestimated.

### *Example 5.1*

Hsieh (1988) reported on the results of a pilot study for a planned 5-year trial examining cardiovascular risk factors. Cholesterol levels (mg/dl) were obtained from 754 individuals from four worksites. The estimated value of the variance component within worksites is given by $S_W^2 = 2209$, while that between worksites is given by $S_A^2 = 93$. Therefore the value of the intracluster correlation coefficient may be assessed for the purpose of sample size estimation as

$$\rho = \frac{93}{(93 + 2209)} = \frac{93}{2302} = 0.04$$

Assuming approximately 70 eligible subjects per worksite, this implies that the variance inflation factor is given by $1 + (70 - 1)0.04 = 3.76$. The number of worksites which must be randomized to obtain 80 per cent power at $\alpha = 0.05$ (two-sided) for detecting a mean difference in cholesterol level of 20 mg/dl between intervention groups is then given by

$$k = \frac{(1.96 + 0.84)^2\, 2(2302)[1 + (70 - 1)0.04]}{70(20^2)} = 4.8$$

In practice, at least seven clusters might be randomly assigned per intervention group both to adjust for the use of critical values corresponding to the normal rather than the $t$-distribution and to allow for the possibility that one or two worksites might not participate for the full length of the trial. Then a total of 490 subjects would need to be recruited to each intervention group, assuming 70 subjects recruited per worksite and seven worksites per intervention group. Due to observed between-worksite variation in cholesterol levels, however, this sample size is effectively equivalent to an individually randomized trial with 130 subjects in each intervention group ($130 \simeq 490/3.76$). Any final determination of sample size should also consider a range of plausible values for both $\rho$ and $\sigma^2$, especially since the pilot study was limited to only four worksites. For example, if the true intracluster correlation $\rho = 0.10$, the variance inflation factor would be $1 + (70 - 1)0.10 = 7.9$, yielding $k = 10.2$.

### *Further remarks*

1. As noted by several authors (e.g. Koepsell *et al.* 1991, Murray and Short 1995) some improvement in power for cohort studies may almost always be obtained by taking into account the proportion of variation explained in the outcome measure by one or more baseline covariates. A natural choice for this purpose is the pre-test version of a post-test outcome measure.

   To account for the influence of a single covariate in the calculation of sample size, the value $(1 - r^2)\sigma^2$ could be substituted for $\sigma^2$ in equation (5.1), where $r$ is the anticipated correlation, possibly based on previous data, between the covariate and the outcome measure. For example, if $r = 0.5$, the required sample size may be reduced by 25 per cent, a saving which may be particularly attractive when resources are limited.

Adjustment for covariates measured at the cluster level (e.g. cluster size) should reduce the between-cluster source of variation and hence also reduce the value of $\rho$. In general this should also lead to an increase in power, depending on the relationship between the covariate and the outcome measure. This reflects the point made in Section 5.1, where, in considering the effect of stratification on the value of $\rho$, it was assumed that the strata are defined at the cluster level. However, the situation is more complicated when adjusting for baseline covariates measured at the individual level (e.g. age, sex). Increased power due to covariate adjustment may then be accompanied by either an increase or a decrease in the size of $\rho$. A more detailed discussion of the effect of covariate adjustment on the value of the intracluster correlation is provided by Stanish and Taylor (1983).

To account for the influence of several baseline covariates, the multiple correlation coefficient $R$ replaces $r$ in this expression, as illustrated by Murray and Short (1995). However, in many applications a suitable value of $R$ may not be available from empirical sources. In this case, it is useful to note that application of the relatively simple formula (5.1) will be conservative, i.e. it will tend to overestimate the actual required trial size.

Aside from increasing precision, recording a pre-test version of a post-test measure has the additional advantage of providing baseline data that can be used to reassess the values of $\sigma_A^2$, $\sigma_W^2$ and $\rho$, thus providing a check on the validity of sample size calculations that may rely heavily on the assumed values of these parameters.

2. In some trials, it may be considered more natural to frame the scientific question of interest in terms of a subject's change score from baseline rather than in terms of the final score alone. The primary analysis would then consist of comparing the average change in the experimental group with the corresponding average change in the control group. Assuming that the variation in the baseline and final scores is the same, the variance of a change score is given by $2\sigma^2(1-r)$, where $r$ again denotes the correlation between the two scores. Then the appropriate size of sample is obtained by substituting $2\sigma^2(1-r)$ for $\sigma^2$ in equation (5.1). This shows that it is statistically more efficient to compare the net changes in baseline between the two groups than it is to compare the final scores alone provided $r > 0.5$ (Fleiss 1986, Section 7.1). Note also that in this case the value of $\rho$ in equation (5.1) technically corresponds to the change score rather than the final score.
3. Although assignment of an equal number of clusters per intervention group is usually most efficient from a statistical perspective, practical considerations may occasionally suggest unequal allocation, as, for example, was done in the CATCH (Zucker *et al.* 1995). In this case, formula (5.2) may be easily adopted to calculate the required total sample size. Denoting the number of clusters to be enrolled in the experimental group by $k_1$, suppose we wish to enrol $k_2 = Qk_1$ clusters in the control group. Then to preserve the same error rate specifications as obtained under equal allocation with $k$ clusters per group ($Q = 1$), the numbers of clusters required under unequal allocation are given approximately by

$$k_1 = \tfrac{1}{2}k(1 + 1/Q) \qquad \text{and} \qquad k_2 = \tfrac{1}{2}k(1 + Q)$$

As would be expected, it can be easily shown that $K = k_1 + k_2$ exceeds $2k$, the total number of clusters required under equal allocation, where the increment

$K - 2k$ may be viewed as the sample size penalty imposed by the unequal allocation scheme. Furthermore, the number of additional clusters needed to achieve the same trial power as obtained under equal allocation will steadily increase with the allocation ratio $Q$. Thus, in practice, the selected value of $Q$ will rarely exceed 2 or 3, since the resulting loss of power may then become prohibitive.

4. The discussion above focuses on the case of comparing two means. Sample size and power considerations for the comparison of two or more means using an analysis of variance framework have been discussed by Koepsell *et al.* (1991) and Feldman and McKinlay (1994). This framework also allows the investigator to take into account anticipated time trends that may be associated with the intervention in either longitudinal studies or studies involving repeated cross-sectional samples. Inferences can then be conducted that focus on a comparison between the experimental and control groups with respect to the pattern of change over time.

## 5.2.2 Subsample size and statistical efficiency

It was mentioned in Section 5.1 that some cluster randomization trials are designed to enrol only a sample of eligible cluster members, i.e. to adopt a subsampling strategy. In this section we consider the implications of subsampling for study planning.

The effect of subsample size on statistical efficiency is most easily understood using a design framework in which the unit of randomization has been selected and a method identified for sampling subjects. These conditions imply that increasing the subsample size affects the precision with which the intracluster correlation coefficient is estimated, but not its underlying value. For purposes of sample size determination, statistical efficiency can then be assessed for different fixed values of $\rho$ while varying the number of clusters per intervention group, $k$, and the subsample size, $m$. Although attention here is limited to quantitative outcomes and completely randomized designs, analogous results may be derived for other outcomes and experimental designs.

It is interesting to examine the relative effect on power of increasing the number of clusters versus increasing the subsample size. The variance of the mean difference $\overline{Y}_1 - \overline{Y}_2$ as computed over all study participants is given by

$$\operatorname{Var}(\overline{Y}_1 - \overline{Y}_2) = \frac{2\sigma^2}{km}[1 + (m-1)\rho] \tag{5.3}$$

It is clear from this expression that as $k$ becomes large, $\operatorname{Var}(\overline{Y}_1 - \overline{Y}_2)$ approaches zero, implying that the power of the study may be increased indefinitely by recruiting more clusters. However, as $m$ becomes large with the number of clusters fixed, $\operatorname{Var}(\overline{Y}_1 - \overline{Y}_2)$ approaches $(2\sigma^2\rho)/k = 2\sigma_A^2/k$, showing that power may be improved by increasing the subsample size only to an upper bound which is limited by the value of $\sigma_A^2$. After this bound is reached, $\operatorname{Var}(\overline{Y}_1 - \overline{Y}_2)$ becomes almost totally dominated by $\sigma_A^2$, implying that the power for testing the effect of intervention will then become largely insensitive to the value of $m$, as explicitly demonstrated by Hsieh (1988).

Inspection of equation (5.3) makes it clear that up to a point, the same level of precision for estimating the effect of intervention may be achieved by choosing different values of $m$ and $k$. In some trials, the value of $m$ will be effectively fixed by practical considerations. However, at times there may be an opportunity to increase $k$ at the expense of $m$, or possibly vice versa. In making this choice, Thompson *et al.* (1997b) caution against reducing the number of clusters, $k$, and increasing the subsample size $m$ simply on statistical grounds. This is because reducing the number of clusters randomized limits the generalizability of the results 'either in fact or as perceived by others'. An additional cautionary factor is that there is generally much greater uncertainty concerning the likely value of $\sigma_A^2$ than there is concerning $\sigma_W^2$, implying that a strategy of allowing $\sigma_A^2$ to almost totally dominate the precision of the study may not be prudent. Thus, from a statistical perspective, increasing the number of clusters while reducing the average subsample size will often be the preferred strategy. This may be difficult from a practical perspective, however, since the number of available clusters may be sharply limited by cost or other constraints in the field (Kelder *et al.* 1993, Hayes 1998).

Although its impact on trial power will usually be deleterious, the decision is sometimes made to recruit clusters of relatively large size, even at the expense of the total number of clusters enrolled. This decision could be made in part to avoid logistical or ethical problems that may otherwise arise. For example, in the REACT (Rapid Early Action for Coronary Treatment) study, the intervention was designed to reduce the delay between onset of symptoms or acute myocardial infarction and patients' arrival at a hospital emergency department (Feldman *et al.* 1998). These investigators, although recognizing that reducing the sample size per community would not have a serious impact on power, stated that this option

> was not practical in REACT and would not necessarily have lowered the cost of the trial, because the fixed expense of maintaining data-collection staff and conducting the intervention in additional communities might have outweighed any savings in volume of cases.

Suppose the number of clusters available to the investigators cannot exceed a specified maximum value, as determined by cost constraints or other practical considerations, but that some control is nevertheless retained over the subsample size. Then it may be most convenient to specify the sample size requirements in terms of the number of subjects required per cluster. Let $k_{max}$ denote the maximum number of clusters which can be assigned per intervention group. One can then show that the number of subjects required per cluster is given by the equation

$$m = (1-\rho)\Big/\left(\frac{k_{max}}{k_{(m=1)}} - \rho\right) \qquad (5.4)$$

where

$$k_{(m=1)} = \frac{(t_{\alpha/2} + t_\beta)^2(2\sigma^2)}{(\mu_1 - \mu_2)^2}$$

denotes the number of clusters per intervention group which would be required if $m = 1$. Justification for equation (5.4) is based on solving the equation $k_{max}/k_{(m=1)} = [1 + (m-1)\rho]/m$ for the subsample size $m$ (Hsieh 1988), where $t$ has $2(k_{max} - 1)$ degrees of freedom. Note the restriction imposed by these algebraic relationships that the value of $\rho$ used to select the subsample size must be less than $k_{max}/k_{(m=1)}$. The use here of critical values corresponding to the $t$-distribution rather than the normal distribution is particularly important for trials in which $k_{max}$ is small.

We illustrate application of equation (5.4) by revisiting the worksite intervention trial discussed previously in Example 5.1 (Hsieh 1988). This trial was designed to detect a difference in mean cholesterol levels across intervention groups of 20 mg/dl, using data from a pilot study indicating that $\sigma^2$ may be assessed as 2302 and $\rho$ as 0.04. Suppose the trial investigators were limited to recruiting $k_{max} = 6$ clusters per intervention group. Since

$$k_{(m=1)} = \frac{(2.228 + 0.879)^2\, 2(2302)}{20^2} = 111$$

the required subsample size at $\alpha = 0.05$ (two-sided) and $1 - \beta = 0.80$ is given by

$$m = (1 - 0.04) \bigg/ \left(\frac{6}{111} - 0.04\right) = 69$$

Accordingly, if only six worksites are included per intervention group, at least 69 subjects will need to be sampled per worksite to achieve the desired power, a result which is similar to that obtained in Example 5.1.

## 5.2.3 Comparison of proportions

We may use the same approach as adopted in Section 5.2.1 to obtain sample size requirements for comparing two rates or proportions in a cluster randomization trial. Assume again that $k$ clusters of $m$ individuals each are randomly assigned to each group $i$ ($i = 1, 2$), where $i = 1$ denotes the experimental group and $i = 2$ denotes the control group. The aim of the investigators is to test the hypothesis $H_0 : P_1 = P_2$ at the two-sided $100\alpha$ per cent level of significance with power $1 - \beta$, where $P_1$ and $P_2$ are the population success rates in the experimental and control groups, respectively. Sample estimates of $P_1$ and $P_2$ are given by $\hat{P}_1$ and $\hat{P}_2$, respectively, where these estimates are computed over all individuals in each group.

Let $Z_{\alpha/2}$, $Z_\beta$ again denote the critical values of the standard normal distribution corresponding to the error rates $\alpha$ and $\beta$, respectively. Then the required number of subjects per intervention group is given approximately by

$$n = \frac{(Z_{\alpha/2} + Z_\beta)^2 [P_1(1 - P_1) + P_2(1 - P_2)][1 + (m - 1)\rho]}{(P_1 - P_2)^2} \qquad (5.5)$$

and thus the required number of clusters per group by $k = n/m$.

At $\rho = 0$, equation (5.5) reduces to the standard sample size specification for comparing two proportions (e.g. Pocock 1983, Section 9.1). The inflation factor $IF = 1 + (m - 1)\rho$ may also be applied to other versions of this sample size formulation, given, for example, by Armitage and Berry (1994, Section 6.6) and Cohen (1988, Section 10.6).

Cornfield (1978) took a different approach to developing an equivalent expression for sample size estimation. The primary difference is that the inflation factor is calculated as the ratio of two variances. Following Cornfield (1978), suppose that a community intervention trial is being designed to reduce cardiovascular mortality, and we have access to the following annual cardiovascular mortality data (per

100 000) from five US counties: 249, 234, 288, 271, 261. The mean and variance of these annual rates are given by $P = 261$ deaths/100 000 and $\sigma^2 = (21 \text{ deaths}/100\,000)^2$, respectively. However, if the variation in mortality among clusters is ignored, the variance of an individual mortality rate would be given by $P(1 - P)/m$, where $m = 150\,000$ is the mean county population. Recognizing that the variance inflation factor $IF = 1 + (m - 1)\rho$ may be written as the ratio of these two variances, we have

$$IF = \frac{\sigma^2}{P(1 - P)/m}$$

$$= \frac{0.000\,21^2}{0.002\,61(1 - 0.002\,61)/150\,000} = 2.5$$

This result implies that standard sample estimates should be inflated by a factor of 2.5 if the trial is to be designed using cluster randomization.

For studies randomizing a relatively large number of small clusters, explicit formulation of the factor $IF$ in terms of the parameter $\rho$, as illustrated in Example 5.1, will usually be the most practical approach to estimating sample size. However, the version of $IF$ given by Cornfield (1978) seems natural when a relatively small number of large clusters, such as entire communities or counties, are to be randomized, particularly when information on the cluster-specific event rates is readily available. Thus Cornfield's illustration of this approach uses published cardiovascular mortality rates for the five counties that participated in the Stanford Five City community intervention trial (Farquhar 1978). However, the resulting sample size estimate must inevitably suffer from considerable uncertainty, as would be the case for any estimate based on data from such a small number of communities.

### *Example 5.2*

Murray *et al.* (1992) reported on a study evaluating the effect of school-based interventions in reducing adolescent tobacco use. One aspect of this trial involved a comparison of the Smoke Free Generation intervention with the Existing Curriculum on the proportion of children who report using smokeless tobacco after 2 years of follow-up. An estimate of the within-school intracluster correlation coefficient can be calculated from 24 schools, 12 randomized to each intervention group, as 0.01. Suppose a new trial is being designed with approximately 100 students per school, and it is of interest to detect a reduction in the anticipated control group event rate of $P_2 = 0.06$ to a rate of $P_1 = 0.04$, representing a 33 per cent decline. If the comparison is to be performed at the 5 per cent level of significance (two-sided) with 80 per cent power, then the number of individuals to be randomized to each group is obtained from equation (5.5) as

$$n = \frac{(1.96 + 0.84)^2[(0.04)(0.96) + (0.06)(0.94)][1 + (100 - 1)0.01]}{(0.04 - 0.06)^2}$$

$$= 3698$$

In practice, 38 schools might be randomized to each of the two intervention groups to assure that the trial has sufficient power.

### 5.2.4 Comparison of incidence rates

In some studies, the effect of intervention may be measured as the reduction in the incidence rate of a condition, where the denominator of the event rate is the number of person-years of follow-up in the cluster rather than the number of persons. Methods of analysis for such cluster randomization trials have been considered by several investigators (e.g. Moore and Tsiatis 1991, Duffy *et al.* 1992 and Brookmeyer and Chen 1998). All such methods are extensions of better known techniques for the analyses of count or Poisson data, often encountered in the design and analysis of cohort studies (e.g. Breslow and Day 1987). These extensions are characterized by their allowance for between-cluster variation in incidence rates.

Suppose that $k$ clusters are randomly assigned to each group $i$ $(i = 1, 2)$, where $i = 1$ denotes the experimental group, $i = 2$ the control group, and where the members of each cluster are followed for a total of $t$ person-years. The aim of the investigators may be to test the hypothesis $H_0 : \lambda_1 = \lambda_2$ at the two-sided $100\alpha$ per cent level of significance with power $1 - \beta$, where $\lambda_1$ denotes the incidence rate per person-year in the population of experimental group clusters, and $\lambda_2$ denotes the corresponding rate in the control group clusters. We let $\sigma_1^2$ and $\sigma_2^2$ denote the variance components representing between-cluster variation in incidence rates for the experimental and control groups, respectively.

Following Hayes *et al.* (1995) and Hayes and Bennett (1999), we make the simplifying assumption that the coefficient of variation $CV$ is the same across groups, where

$$CV = \sigma_2/\lambda_2 = \sigma_1/\lambda_1$$

The parameter $CV$ defined here plays a similar role to that of the intracluster correlation coefficient in the case of continuous or binary outcome data. Thus larger values of the coefficient of variation indicate greater between-cluster variability, leading to an inflation of the required sample size.

With this formulation, the number of clusters required in each group is given by

$$k = \frac{(Z_{\alpha/2} + Z_\beta)^2(\lambda_1 + \lambda_2)}{t(\lambda_1 - \lambda_2)^2} IF_t \tag{5.6}$$

where

$$IF_t = 1 + \frac{CV^2(\lambda_1^2 + \lambda_2^2)t}{\lambda_1 + \lambda_2}$$

denotes the variance inflation due to clustering. Note that in the absence of between-cluster variation, the coefficient of variation $CV = 0$ and the inflation factor $IF_t = 1$. Equation (5.6) then reduces to standard sample size formulas as used in the design of cohort studies (Hayes and Bennett 1999).

An alternative but algebraically identical expression was provided by Hayes and Bennett (1999). However, these authors recommend allocating $k + 1$ clusters to each intervention group to compensate for the use of the critical values $Z_{\alpha/2}$, $Z_\beta$ in equation (5.6). This is an alternative form of the degrees of freedom correction strategy presented in Section 5.2.1.

In general, it can be seen from equation (5.6) that there is a trade-off between the number of person-years required per cluster and the number of clusters. Moreover, as the coefficient of variation $CV$ increases, there are diminishing returns from increasing the number of person-years. Hence for large clusters, it may be cost-efficient to subsample individuals for follow-up within each cluster (Hayes 1998).

### Example 5.3

Hayes *et al.* (1995) provide an example of how equation (5.6) may be applied to a trial of HIV prevention. Although this was a matched-pair trial, matching was ignored in the estimation of sample size on the grounds that the resulting calculation should be conservative in the presence of effective matching. This is a very reasonable approach, particularly when prior information concerning the likely effectiveness of matching is not available. In this study, $\lambda_2$, the expected incidence of HIV per person-year in the control communities, was assumed to be 0.01. Investigators were interested in reducing the incidence rate from 0.01 to 0.005 cases of HIV per person-year. The assumed common value of the coefficient of variation $CV = \sigma_1/\lambda_1 = \sigma_2/\lambda_2$ was taken to be 0.25.

Application of equation (5.6) shows that a sample of 1000 individuals per community, each followed for 2 years (2000 person-years of observation), will provide 80 per cent power at $\alpha = 0.05$ (two-sided) for detecting a 50 per cent reduction in average HIV incidence from 0.01 to 0.005 HIV cases per person-year provided $k = 5$ communities are enrolled per group. The detailed calculations are as follows:

$$IF_t = 1 + \frac{0.25^2(0.005^2 + 0.01^2)2000}{(0.005 + 0.01)}$$

$$= 2.04$$

$$k = \frac{(1.96 + 0.84)^2(0.005 + 0.01)}{2000(0.005 - 0.01)^2}(2.04)$$

$$= 4.8$$

Ultimately $k + 1 = 6$ communities were enrolled per group to compensate for use of the critical values $Z_{\alpha/2}$, $Z_\beta$ in this calculation.

This example is also noteworthy for the care taken by the investigators in considering a range of plausible values for the parameter $CV$. Hayes and Bennett (1999) provide further discussion on how values of the coefficient of variation may be selected for the purpose of sample size planning.

## 5.3 The matched-pair design

As discussed in Section 3.4, the matched-pair design is one in which each cluster is matched ('paired') with a similar cluster. One cluster in each pair, which we may think of as a stratum, is then randomly assigned to intervention and one to control. This design is therefore distinguished from the completely randomized and stratified designs in that it involves no replication of clusters within any combination of intervention and stratum. Thus estimates of random variability among clusters can only be disentangled from intervention effects by using between-stratum information.

## 5.3.1 Comparison of means

As in Section 5.2.1, we assume that the primary response variable for the trial is denoted by $Y$, where $Y$ is assumed to be normally distributed. Suppose the matched-pair allocation gives rise to the observed mean differences $d_j = \overline{Y}_{1j} - \overline{Y}_{2j}$, $j = 1, 2, \ldots, k$, where $\overline{Y}_{1j}$ and $\overline{Y}_{2j}$ are computed over clusters of size $m_{1j}$ and $m_{2j}$, respectively. We assume that the aim of the investigators is to determine the number of pairs $k$ needed to test $H_0 : \Delta = 0$, where $\Delta$ is the population mean of the $d_j$. For example, investigators in the Take Heart trial (Glasgow *et al.* 1995b) matched a heterogeneous sample of worksites with respect to key organizational characteristics and then randomly assigned one worksite in a pair to an early or delayed intervention. The final recruitment of 13 pairs of worksites provided 90 per cent power to detect a mean difference of 10 mg/dl in cholesterol at the two-sided 5 per cent level using a paired $t$-test performed at the cluster level.

Assuming $m_{1j} = m_{2j} = m$, $j = 1, 2, \ldots, k$, the required number of pairs for this design depends on the variance of the $d_j$, given by

$$\mathrm{Var}(d_j) = 2\left(\frac{\sigma_W^2}{m} + \sigma_{AM}^2\right) \tag{5.7}$$

where $\sigma_W^2$ denotes the within-cluster component of variability and $\sigma_{AM}^2$ denotes the component of variability between the two clusters in a matched pair (Thompson *et al.* 1997b). The subscript $\sigma_{AM}^2$ is used here to distinguish $\sigma_{AM}^2$ from $\sigma_A^2$, the between-cluster variance component for a completely randomized design. Provided the matching is effective, $\sigma_{AM}^2$ will be reduced in value as compared with $\sigma_A^2$, perhaps substantially. With this formulation, the number of pairs required to test $H_0$ at the two-sided $100\alpha$ per cent level of significance with power $1 - \beta = 0.80$ is given by

$$k = \frac{(Z_{\alpha/2} + Z_\beta)^2\,\mathrm{Var}(d_j)}{\Delta^2} \tag{5.8}$$

where $\Delta$ is the minimum difference to be detected.

If $\sigma_{AM}^2$ is estimated from a population of clusters more heterogeneous than the clusters within a matched-pair, then the sample size estimate above will be conservative. This may well be the only option available, given that investigators are forced to rely in practice on whatever data are both accessible and relevant to their purpose. The overall task is clearly simplified if relevant information on $\mathrm{Var}(d_j)$ is directly available from a previously conducted trial.

An alternative version of this result is obtained by multiplying equation (5.2), which provides the required number of clusters per group for a completely randomized design, by the factor $1 - \rho_M$, where $\rho_M$ denotes the correlation between $\overline{Y}_{1j}$ and $\overline{Y}_{2j}$. Following Freedman *et al.* (1990), the relative efficiency of the matched pair to the completely randomized design, ignoring differences in the degrees of freedom, may be defined as $1/(1 - \rho_M)$. Thus if an unmatched design requires $2k$ clusters to ensure adequate statistical power, then $2k(1 - \rho_M)$ clusters would be required using the matched design, a reduction of $100(1 - \rho_M)$ per cent in the required sample size. The parameter $\rho_M$, which directly measures the effectiveness of the pairing, was referred to in Section 3.6 as the 'matching correlation'. It is clear that if prior information on $\rho_M$ is not available, a conservative strategy is simply to set $\rho_M = 0$, i.e. use equation (5.2) to plan the size of the trial.

As with the completely randomized design, use of the critical values $Z_{\alpha/2}$, $Z_\beta$ in equation (5.8) rather than critical values from a $t$-distribution will underestimate the required sample size unless the degrees of freedom are large. The addition of two more pairs of clusters is sufficient to adjust for this undercorrection when the sample size is determined using a 5 per cent type I error rate (Snedecor and Cochran 1989, p. 104). Three additional pairs of clusters should be added to approximate the critical values from a $t$-distribution when a 1 per cent type I error rate is used. However, no such correction is needed when 30 or more pairs of clusters are being randomized (Lachin 1981).

### *Example 5.4*

The purpose of the British Family Heart Study (Thompson *et al.* 1997b) was to estimate the effect of a cardiovascular and health screening examination on the development of subsequent coronary risk factors. Thirteen pairs of practices were selected from the same town, based on the similarity of their patient populations with respect to a number of demographic and social characteristics, as well as their willingness to be randomized.

The sample size for the trial was chosen on the basis of what the authors describe as a precision-based rather than a power-based criterion. This criterion assured that the standard error of the mean cholesterol difference between the experimental and control groups was less than a pre-specified value. From equation (5.7), the standard error of $\bar{d} = \sum_{j=1}^{k} d_j/k$ is obtained as

$$\mathrm{SE}(\bar{d}) = \sqrt{\frac{2}{k}\left(\frac{\sigma_W^2}{m} + \sigma_{AM}^2\right)}$$

As discussed above, it is usually much more difficult to anticipate a realistic value for $\sigma_{AM}^2$ than for $\sigma_W^2$. Nonetheless the investigators were able to obtain a rough estimate of $\sigma_{AM}^2$ for a number of coronary risk factors by taking advantage of a previously published study. The previous study presented mean risk factor levels in 40–59 year-old men from a single general practice in each of 24 towns, data which could be used to obtain advance estimates of both $\sigma_W^2$ and $\sigma_{AM}^2$. The values of these variance components for serum cholesterol were estimated to be $\sigma_W^2 = 1.0$ mmol/l and $\sigma_{AM}^2 = 0.01$ mmol/l, allowing $\mathrm{SE}(\bar{d})$ to be tabulated as a function of the number of clusters, $k$, and the number of patients per practice. On the basis of a series of such calculations, the investigators chose to recruit 200 men from each of two practices in each of 15 towns, ensuring that $\mathrm{SE}(\bar{d})$ would be no greater than 0.045. Although other combinations of $(m, k)$, such as $(100, 20)$ or $(50, 30)$, would also achieve this level of precision, the final selection of 15 pairs was determined, as is inevitably the case, by issues of feasibility and funding. Thirteen of these pairs were ultimately enrolled in the trial.

## 5.3.2 Comparison of proportions

Let $m_{1j}$, $m_{2j}$ denote the sizes of the clusters randomized to the experimental and control interventions, respectively $(j = 1, 2, \ldots, k)$. The allocation scheme associated with this design gives rise to the observed sample differences $d_j = \hat{P}_{1j} - \hat{P}_{2j}$, where $\hat{P}_{1j}$ and $\hat{P}_{2j}$ estimate the true event rates $P_{1j}$, $P_{2j}$. Our aim is to determine the number of pairs, $k$, required to test $H_0 : \Delta = 0$, where $\Delta$ is the population mean of the $d_j$. This will be done under the assumption that a paired $t$-test is to be performed on the $d_j$, although other approaches to the analysis may also be taken, such as Fisher's non-parametric permutation test (Gail *et al.* 1992, Green 1997). Unlike the paired $t$-test, this approach involves no distributional assumptions on the $d_j$, obtained at the price of some loss in power. However, the two procedures are asymptotically equivalent, justifying the use of the paired $t$-test in estimating the required sample size.

The required number of the pairs for the trial depends on the variance of $d_j$, given approximately by

$$\mathrm{Var}(d_j) = \frac{P_{1j}(1 - P_{1j})}{m_{1j}} + \frac{P_{2j}(1 - P_{2j})}{m_{2j}} + 2\sigma^2_{\mathrm{AM}}$$

where the first two terms of this expression represent the usual binomial variation within clusters (governed in part by the cluster sizes) and $\sigma^2_{\mathrm{AM}}$ is the between-cluster variance component (Thompson *et al.* 1997b). The quantity $\sigma^2_{\mathrm{AM}}$ may be regarded as measuring the inherent variability between two clusters in a matched pair that exists in the absence of an intervention effect. For the purposes of sample size estimation, it is reasonable to replace $P_{1j}$ and $P_{2j}$ by their anticipated mean values, $P_1$ and $P_2$, respectively, and to set $m_{1j} = m_{2j} = m$.

The number of pairs needed to achieve power $1 - \beta$ for detecting a difference $\Delta$ at the two-sided $100\alpha$ per cent significance level is then given by

$$k = (Z_{\alpha/2} + Z_{\beta})^2 \frac{\mathrm{Var}(d_j)}{\Delta^2} \tag{5.9}$$

This formula, as usual, does not take into account that a $t$-statistic based on $k - 1$ degrees of freedom, rather than a standard normal deviate test, will be used to test $H_0$. Allowance for the degrees of freedom may be obtained by using the same adjustments described earlier in Section 5.3.1.

### *Example 5.5*

Gail *et al.* (1992) and Green (1997) described the sample size approach used for the COMMIT trial, where the primary outcome variable was the difference in smoking quit rates between the experimental and control communities. The statistic of interest was $d_j = \hat{P}_{1j} - \hat{P}_{2j}$, where $\hat{P}_{1j}$ is the estimate of the quit rate for the experimental community in pair $j$, and $\hat{P}_{2j}$ the corresponding estimate for the control community.

It is interesting to note that this trial was one of the first community randomized studies to use formal statistical considerations in estimating the required sample size. A possibly related consequence was that the eventual size of this study was more than triple that of previously reported community intervention trials on smoking cessation (Freedman *et al.* 1997).

The basic approach adopted by these investigators was to use equation (5.9) to calculate the number of community pairs required under the assumption that each community will supply a cohort of $m$ subjects. Then the variance of the $d_j$ may be written

$$\mathrm{Var}(d_j) = \frac{P_1(1 - P_1) + P_2(1 - P_2)}{m} + 2\sigma^2_{\mathrm{AM}}$$

where $P_1$, $P_2$ are the true quit rates in the experimental and control groups, respectively, and $\sigma^2_{\text{AM}}$ represents the component of variability between two communities in a matched pair. Since there was some uncertainty regarding the value of $\sigma^2_{\text{AM}}$, various sensitivity analyses were carried out to determine the effect of different values of this parameter on the estimated study size. Gail *et al.* (1992), using quit rates from a previous study on smoking cessation, estimated $2\sigma^2_{\text{AM}}$ as 0.006 36.

The sample size strategy used here was conservative, inasmuch as the previous study did not use a matched design. Suppose the smoking quit rate in the control group is $P_2 = 0.15$, and it is of interest to detect an increase in this rate to $P_1 = 0.25$ in the experimental group. Taking the cluster size $m$ as 500 and ignoring allowance for the degrees of freedom, the required number of pairs may be calculated from equation (5.9) at $\alpha = 0.05$ (one-sided) and $1 - \beta = 0.90$ as $k \simeq 6$. It is also interesting to note that the between-community component of variation contributes much more heavily to this result than the binomial component, a consequence of the large number of subjects selected per cluster. As implemented, COMMIT actually recruited 11 pairs of communities, with approximately 550 heavy smokers in each.

### 5.3.3 Comparison of incidence rates

Suppose now that the outcome of interest in a matched-pair trial is the incidence rate of a condition. For example, Stanton and Clemens (1987) report on a matched-pair community intervention trial examining the effect of a water-sanitation education programme on childhood diarrhoea rates (per 100 person-weeks). As a second example, Ray *et al.* (1997) discuss a randomized trial of a consultation service to reduce the rate of injurious falls (per 100 person-years) among residents of 14 paired nursing homes.

As noted in Section 5.2.4, a conservative estimate of sample size for such trials may be obtained using equation (5.6), an approach which ignores the pairing. The assessment of sample size then requires specification of the parameter $CV$, the coefficient of variation in incidence rates, assumed to be fixed across intervention groups.

More accurate estimates of the required sample size may be determined if relevant data from previous matched-pair trials are available. In this case, the number of required pairs may be determined using equation (5.6) with $CV$ replaced by $CV_{\text{M}}$, the coefficient of variation in incidence rates between clusters within a matched pair. Guidelines that may be used to derive values for $CV_{\text{M}}$ are given by Hayes and Bennett (1999).

We now suppose that each cluster contributes a total of $t$ units of follow-up. Then, under assumptions given by Hayes and Bennett (1999), one can show that $CV_M = CV(1 - \rho_M)$, where $\rho_{\text{M}}$ denotes the correlation between the true incidence rates in the experimental and control clusters in the $i$th matched pair, $i = 1, \ldots, k$. This formulation may be used as an alternative to calculating $CV_{\text{M}}$ directly. It may also be used to demonstrate an equivalence between the approach described by Hayes and Bennett (1999) and an earlier approach described by Shipley *et al.* (1989). Modest differences in required sample size may still result from these two approaches as a result of the different methods used to correct for degrees of freedom.

## 5.4 The stratified design

Lachin and Bautista (1995) have investigated the benefit gained from taking into account stratification in planning the sample size for trials randomizing individuals. Their results show that stratification by baseline covariates may be safely ignored for this purpose unless the covariate response association is sizeable and there is considerable covariate imbalance. However, the smaller effective sample size associated with cluster randomization implies that the probability of imbalance on important prognostic factors will, in general, tend to be greater than in designs which randomize individuals to intervention groups. Therefore, accounting for stratification in the estimation of sample size may also be more important for such designs, particularly when the number of randomized clusters is small.

### 5.4.1 Comparison of means

The stratified design can be regarded as a replication of the completely randomized design as implemented separately in each of $S$ strata, where the strata are defined by cluster-level variables measured at baseline. The main impact of stratification on the assessment of sample size for testing the equality of means with respect to a quantitative response variable is obtained through the corresponding reduction obtained in $\sigma_A^2$, the between-cluster variance component of the overall response variance $\sigma^2$. From the perspective of trial power, this variance component may now be taken as the residual variance among clusters within strata. The actual gain in precision resulting from stratification will often be difficult to judge in advance. However, this gain will always be positive if the stratification is effective and the degrees of freedom are large ($\geqslant 30$, say). In this case, a conservative strategy would be to ignore this aspect of the design in sample size planning.

### 5.4.2 Comparison of proportions

In stratified designs with a dichotomous outcome, it is convenient analytically to express the effect of intervention through its impact on the relative odds (odds ratio) of a successful outcome. However, the assumption of a common odds ratio from stratum to stratum is more complicated from the perspective of sample size estimation than is the assumption of a common difference in means or in rates. This is because the value of a common odds ratio will, in general, differ from the value of the crude odds ratio which characterizes the effect of intervention obtained while ignoring stratification. We also note that this issue is closely related to the observation of Hauck *et al.* (1998) that, for analyses with linear models, covariate adjustment is a precision issue only, while for non-linear analyses the intervention effect which is estimated also changes with such adjustment.

Let $P_{1j}$ and $P_{2j}, j = 1, 2, \ldots, S$, denote the anticipated stratum-specific success rates in the experimental and control groups, respectively. We assume that the value of the intervention odds ratio

$$\Psi = \frac{P_{1j}(1 - P_{2j})}{P_{2j}(1 - P_{1j})}$$

is constant across strata, implying

$$P_{1j} = \frac{P_{2j}\Psi}{1 - P_{2j} + P_{2j}\Psi} \tag{5.10}$$

Let $\overline{P}_j = (P_{1j} + P_{2j})/2$ denote the overall success rate for stratum $j, j = 1, 2, \ldots, S$, and let $f_j$ denote the fraction of individuals in the trial belonging to stratum $j$, where $\sum_{j=1}^{S} f_j = 1$. Assuming that $n_j$ clusters, each of size $m_j$, are allocated in balanced fashion to each intervention group within stratum $j$, the total number of subjects required for testing $H_0 : \Psi = 1$ is given (e.g. Donner 1998) by

$$N = \frac{(Z_{\alpha/2}T + Z_{\beta}U)^2}{V^2} \tag{5.11}$$

where

$$T = \frac{1}{2}\sqrt{\sum_{j=1}^{S} f_j[1 + (m_j - 1)\rho][\overline{P}_j(1 - \overline{P}_j)]}$$

$$U = \sqrt{\frac{1}{8}\sum_{j=1}^{S} f_j[1 + (m_j - 1)\rho][P_{1j}(1 - P_{1j}) + P_{2j}(1 - P_{2j})]}$$

$$V = \frac{1}{4}\sum_{j=1}^{S} f_j(P_{1j} - P_{2j})$$

and $Z_{\alpha/2}$, $Z_{\beta}$ denote the critical values of the standard normal distribution corresponding to the error rates $\alpha$ and $\beta$.

The parameter $\rho$ is the intracluster correlation coefficient, which we assume constant across strata for the purpose of sample size estimation. The proportion of subjects in the $j$th stratum is then given by $f_j = 2n_jm_j/N$. Since $N = \sum 2n_jm_j$, the number of clusters to be assigned within stratum $j$ to each intervention group is then given by $n_j = (Nf_j)/(2m_j)$. This formula allows the allocation of either a constant number of subjects to each stratum ($f_j = f, j = 1, 2, \ldots, S$) or a constant number of clusters

$$f_j = \frac{m_j}{\sum_j m_j} \quad \text{or} \quad n_j = n = \frac{N}{2\sum_j m_j}$$

The decision to adopt a design in which the number of subjects rather than the number of clusters remains constant from stratum to stratum will usually depend on cost or feasibility factors. However, the use of equation (5.11) for planning purposes is complicated by the need for advance knowledge not only of $\rho$ but also of the stratum-specific success rates $P_{2j}, j = 1, 2, \ldots, S$. This information will sometimes be available from previous studies or other external sources. Alternatively, the choice of strata, and thus of the spacing of the $P_{2j}$, may occasionally be under the control of the investigator. In this case it seems reasonable to assume, at least in terms of the approximations commonly adopted for sample size assessment, that the $P_{2j}$ are equally spaced, say between $P_{21}$ and $P_{2S}$. This implies that $P_{2j} = P_{2(j-1)} + d$, $j = 2, 3, \ldots, S$, where $d = (P_{2S} - P_{21})/(S - 1)$. A prudent strategy in practice would be to compute the required value of $N$ over a series of plausible parameter values in order to ascertain its stability across a variety of underlying assumptions.

This sample size estimation procedure corresponds to application of the well-known Mantel–Haenszel test to the resulting set of $S$ $2 \times 2$ contingency tables (Mantel and Haenszel 1959), suitably adjusted for clustering. The adjusted Mantel–Haenszel test is discussed in Section 6.4.

If the numbers of subjects per cluster is fixed (i.e. $m_j = m$, $j = 1, 2, \ldots, S$), the required sample size $N$ reduces to the expression given by Woolson *et al.* (1986) multiplied by the variance inflation factor $[1 + (m - 1)\rho]$. This expression also reduces approximately to the sample size required for a completely randomized design (see equation 5.5) if there is only a single stratum ($S = 1$).

## Example 5.6

Villar *et al.* (1998) report on a planned cluster randomization trial for the evaluation of a new antenatal care programme. Antenatal care clinics were the natural unit of randomization for this study, not only for administrative and logistical convenience, but also to reduce the experimental contamination that is likely to occur under individual randomization. To further reduce the risk of contamination, only clinics serving distinct neighbourhoods were included. The main purpose of this equivalence trial, conducted across four countries (Thailand, Argentina, Cuba and Saudi Arabia) was to compare the impact of two programmes of antenatal care on the health of mothers and newborns. One of the programmes consists of the 'best standard treatment' (control intervention) as presently offered in antenatal care clinics, with the experimental intervention consisting only of tests, clinical activities and follow-up actions scientifically demonstrated to be effective in improving outcomes (Villar and Bergsjo 1997).

The primary fetal outcome for the study was defined as the rate of low birthweight (<2500 g). The final sample size estimate took into account that the design involved four sites (strata), with antenatal care clinics within each site randomly assigned to an experimental or control group. Further stratification by clinic size, done principally to ensure balanced allocation across intervention groups, was ignored for this purpose.

Given the increased cost and complexity of the 'best standard treatment' relative to the new programme, it was of interest to detect if the odds ratio $\Psi$ associated with the new programme was no more than 1.2, representing an increase in the rate of an adverse outcome (i.e. low birthweight). The value 1.2 was chosen as the maximum value of $\Psi$ that would be regarded as consistent with the conclusion that the new programme is as 'equally effective' as the standard programme, taking into account the increased costs and logistics associated with the latter. Since it was regarded as important to rule out a difference greater than this with high probability, a power of 90 per cent was selected for detecting this effect at the two-sided 5 per cent significance level. Preliminary data from one study site in the trial was used to provide an advance estimate of the intracluster (within-clinic) correlation $\rho$ as 0.000 65. Given

**Table 5.2** Anticipated risk of low birthweight by stratum at $\Psi = 1.2$

| Stratum $j$ | New programme $P_{1j}$ | Best standard treatment $P_{2j}$ | Average $\overline{P}_j$ |
|---|---|---|---|
| 1 | 0.082 84 | 0.07 | 0.076 42 |
| 2 | 0.106 09 | 0.09 | 0.098 05 |
| 3 | 0.129 16 | 0.11 | 0.119 58 |
| 4 | 0.152 05 | 0.13 | 0.141 02 |

the potential instability associated with empirical estimates of the intracluster correlation coefficient, sample size requirements were also calculated for various other plausible values of this parameter.

Assuming a constant number of clinics per stratum, with fixed clinic sizes $m$ taken as 300, 450 or 600 (i.e. $f_j = 1/4$), the sample size requirements for the design were calculated for various values of the intervention odds ratio $\Psi$ (1.16, 1.18, 1.20). Anticipated stratum-specific adverse event rates in the control group $P_{2j}$ were taken to be equally spaced from 0.07 to 0.13, with the $P_{1j}$ obtained from equation (5.10). These are provided in Table 5.2 separately by stratum and intervention group assuming a constant odds ratio of $\Psi = 1.2$.

If $\rho$ is assumed to be 0.001, and $m_j = m = 450$ patients are recruited in each clinic, application of formula (5.11) to the design described shows that the total required sample size is given by

$$N = \frac{[(Z_{0.025}T) + (Z_{0.10}U)]^2}{V^2}$$

$$= \frac{[(1.96)(0.186\,83) + (1.28)(0.186\,75)]^2}{0.004\,3835^2} = 19\,063$$

where

$$T = \frac{1}{2}\sqrt{\sum_{j=1}^{4} f_j[1 + (m_j - 1)\rho][\overline{P}_j(1 - \overline{P}_j)]}$$

$$= 0.186\,83$$

$$U = \sqrt{\frac{1}{8}\sum_{j=1}^{4} f_j[1 + (m_j - 1)\rho][P_{1j}(1 - P_{1j}) + P_{2j}(1 - P_{2j})]} = 0.186\,75$$

and

$$V = \frac{1}{4}\sum_{j=1}^{4} f_j(P_{1j} - P_{2j}) = 0.004\,3835$$

Therefore if $m = 450$ patients are recruited per clinic at least 11 clinics (19 063/[(4)(450)]) would need to be recruited in each of the four specified strata. Ultimately a total of 53 clinics were enrolled in the trial, with a minimum of 12 clinics per site.

An alternative approach to estimating sample size for equivalence trials is to take a confidence interval perspective. Further details of this approach in the context of the antenatal trial are provided by Donner (1998).

## 5.5 Issues involving losses to follow-up

The possibility of loss to follow-up is potentially serious in all randomized trials, but can be a particularly severe problem in cluster randomization trials having a relatively long follow-up time. As noted by Feldman and McKinlay (1994), a loss to follow-up of 5 per cent per year in a cohort of subjects measured at baseline reduces the size of the cohort by nearly 25 per cent in 5 years. For trials in which the interventions are applied at the cluster level, with little or no attention given to individual study participants, the overall attrition rate may well exceed this. Thus some investigators have deliberately adopted an oversampling strategy to help compensate for such losses, followed by aggressive follow-up of those subjects leaving their cluster.

Aside from the risk of loss to follow-up associated with individual subjects, cluster randomization trials must also deal with the possibility that entire clusters may drop out. For example, if there are problems with industrial relations at a particular work-site, all workers at that site may be lost to follow-up. Similarly, the decision of a single administrator may lead to the loss of an entire school in an educational trial. Provided the reasons for loss to follow-up are not related to intervention, oversampling at base-line will help to compensate for both types of losses. Randomizing more clusters than are formally required to detect a specified intervention effect also allows for the inevitable uncertainty associated with the prior assessment of parameters needed for the application of sample size formulas, formulas that in any event must be treated as approximate. This approach was taken by Gail *et al.* (1992) for the COMMIT trial, who generated a range of sample size estimates, corresponding to various levels of the anticipated intervention effect, different assumptions regarding the expected level of intracluster correlation, and various values for the expected sizes of the participating communities (clusters). The investigators then maintained yearly contact with all study subjects. The CATCH (Zucker *et al.* 1995) also oversampled at baseline, but additionally dealt with the possibility of loss to follow-up by adopting a relatively short follow-up period and recruiting only a limited number of students per school.

The British Family Heart Study, discussed above in Example 5.4, used a particu-larly innovative approach to protect against potential loss to follow-up (due to post-randomization refusal) of entire practices. Since this was a matched-pair trial, the loss of a single practice would effectively mean the loss of both practices in the pair. Given that only 13 pairs of practices were to be recruited, this could present serious problems, relating to both power and interpretation. As a precaution, there-fore, the investigators recruited a sample of subjects from each practice in the experimental group to act as an 'internal control'. This internal control was in addition to the external control provided by the matched practice receiving no inter-vention. The latter, however, remained the primary control group for the trial. This decision was made because of a concern that 'awareness of the potential for lifestyle intervention might spill over from the experimental group to other patients in the same practice, including the internal control group'.

As indicated above, losses to follow-up may create bias in the estimated effect of intervention if they do not occur randomly with respect to the intervention assigned. Such bias may also result due to non-adherence to the randomization scheme. This problem is most likely to occur when the effectiveness of the intervention depends directly on the subject's active participation, which is characteristic of many cluster randomization trials, particularly those dealing with prevention. As noted by Black (1996), the intervention may then appear to be weak only because of the beliefs and preferences of the particular subjects involved. The review of cluster randomization trials reported by Simpson *et al.* (1995) indicated various problems of this type. For example, in some studies, clusters were reassigned to a different intervention group after randomization for reasons of cost, feasibility or politics, while in other trials clusters did not receive the assigned intervention. In still others, the analysis was not always done by 'intent to treat', i.e. the primary analysis did not include all clusters randomized. Formulas are available in the clinical trial literature (e.g. Lachin 1981) that can be used to adjust sample size estimates under fairly simple models of non-adherence. However, there is clearly no substitute for taking all possible steps to enhance, monitor and verify compliance with the trial protocol on the part of all study participants.

Post-randomization refusals or dropouts on a cluster level represent an extreme form of non-adherence and may require some difficult choices. One course of action sometimes followed is to formally withdraw such clusters from the trial. However, this raises the issue of response bias. Consider, for example, a school-based trial in which the intervention consists of an enriched educational programme. Schools that have been randomized to the control group may express dissatisfaction by either withdrawing from the trial or seeking to apply components of the desired intervention themselves, possibly through the use of other funding sources. This was an anticipated problem in the Emergency School Assistance Program (ESAP), which provided financial aid that was designed to achieve racial desegregation in southern United States school districts (Crain 1973). The evaluation involved recruiting 150 pairs of schools that were eligible for ESAP and randomly designating one school from each pair as a control. The primary endpoints for the trial consisted of various measures of student achievement. Since the investigators were obliged to say 'no' to 150 school principals, it was recognized that a decision rule would have to be adopted to deal with those schools who declined to accept their assignment to the control group. One possibility was to exclude such schools from the trial, while the other was to allow them to receive the intervention (even at the possible expense of project resources) but be counted in the control group for the purposes of analysis. The first course of action would risk bias in an unpredictable direction, since those schools who were dissatisfied enough with their assignment to actively resist it might be different from those who agreed to accept a control group assignment. On the other hand, the second course of action would clearly lead to a dilution of the intervention effect, thus creating bias in a predictable (conservative) direction. The actual amount of this bias could also be predicted provided the proportion of schools resisting assignment could be anticipated in advance. Thus it was reasoned that the first course of action would disrupt the randomization while the second would disrupt the effect of intervention. Given these two alternatives, the investigators wisely arrived at the following rule: 'given a choice between imperfect randomization of the schools in two treatment-control groups and the imperfect allocation of treatment within the two groups, imperfect treatment is much to be preferred over imperfect randomization'. Eighteen schools in this trial did in fact decline an assignment to the control group.

As discussed in Chapter 3, some trials have used a 'wait-list' approach in an attempt to minimize the problem of refusals and dropouts. For example, the World Health Organization partograph trial (WHO Maternal Health and Safe Motherhood Programme 1994) recruited four pairs of hospitals, with one randomly selected hospital in a matched pair assigned a partograph for the management of labour at the time of randomization. At 10 months into the study, the partograph was introduced into the remaining hospitals and thus used in all eight hospitals for the following 5 months. Aside from encouraging the cooperation of those hospitals who might resist an assignment to the control group, this design also provided more extensive follow-up data for evaluating the impact of the intervention on labour management and outcome. As mentioned in Chapter 4, this design may also alleviate ethical concerns that might otherwise arise.

Of course, loss to follow-up is only a problem in cohort studies, i.e. studies that follow the same individuals over a period of time. This is one reason why some authors (e.g. Feldman and McKinlay 1994) believe that a study design involving a series of cross-sectional samples may sometimes be preferable, even though the cohort design is theoretically more powerful. Nonetheless, cross-sectional designs must cope with other complications that may reduce study power. These include the possibility in community-based trials that immigration of new subjects may occur after the initial baseline survey. Systematic out-migration of subjects surveyed at baseline might also be a problem. Further discussion of these issues is provided in Chapter 3.

## 5.6 Strategies for achieving desired power

Even carefully designed trials may be underpowered. There are a number of strategies investigators can consider using in order to reduce this possibility:

1. Subjects who agree to participate in randomized trials are rarely representative of the general population. Similarly, families, schools, worksites, medical practices and communities which agree to participate in cluster randomization trials may also be unrepresentative, thus impairing external validity (Sorensen *et al.* 1998). On the other hand, 'investigator-driven' selection effects in the form of restrictive eligibility criteria can sometimes have a positive impact on trial power and hence on internal validity. This can be accomplished by placing geographic or other relevant restrictions on the clusters to be randomized, thus reducing between-cluster variability. For example, in a smoking cessation trial reported by LaPrelle *et al.* (1992), it was recognized that variation in smoking rates among communities could be a result of regional or demographic differences between the communities. These differences were avoided by selecting only cities in the South-Eastern United States that were similar with respect to racial and educational make-up. Hayes (1998) also describes a trial in which clusters were deliberately selected to be homogeneous in order to enhance power. Of course, the benefits of such a strategy must always be balanced against the corresponding loss of generalizability.
2. The time and expense needed to mount a trial naturally encourages investigators to request large amounts of data from study subjects. However, this might reduce

subject compliance and the subsequent retention rates of both clusters and subjects within clusters. It might also reduce the number of occasions in longitudinal studies on which any information may be obtained. Therefore all data to be collected in the trial should be carefully justified.

3. Enthusiasm for a new disease prevention or health education programme and concern for the limited number of available clusters might result in overestimating the effect of intervention. Realistic estimates of the minimally important effect of intervention are required if trials are to be adequately powered. Similar considerations apply to estimating the likely loss to follow-up rate. Since the loss to follow-up of entire clusters might be particularly devastating to trial power, this possibility might be given special attention, as for example in the British Family Heart Study (Thompson *et al.* 1997b). As described in Section 5.5, this trial recruited an 'internal control group' to serve as a 'back-up' to the primary control group. Other studies have dealt with this problem by creating a 'reserve' of clusters that would be available to be randomized in the event that this became necessary to preserve the pre-specified level of power.
4. It has been emphasized in this chapter that greater gains in power can be obtained by increasing the number of clusters enrolled than by increasing the number of subjects per cluster. However, it may be administratively or economically difficult to increase the number of clusters assigned to the experimental group beyond some fixed limit. The potential gain in power obtained by increasing the number of clusters assigned to the control group only should then be explored.
5. The primary endpoint for cluster randomization trials is often binary, as when individuals are recorded as either quitting smoking or not. In this case, some gain in power is possible if it is meaningful to expand the definition of such endpoints, e.g. by redefining the smoking variable above as the number of cigarettes smoked per day. Similarly, in cardiovascular trials, the primary endpoint might be expanded to included non-fatal as well as fatal events. Particular care should be taken when dichotomizing continuous endpoints since this can result in a profound loss of power (e.g. Cohen 1983).
6. Cluster randomization trials investigating the effect of intervention on relatively rare events (e.g. death) will need to be quite large in order to be adequately powered. Surrogate endpoints may then be selected to reduce the size and length of the trial. For example, in the antenatal care trial discussed in Example 5.6 (Villar *et al.* 1998), low infant birthweight was used as a surrogate endpoint for perinatal mortality.

   This strategy is only reasonable when the estimated effect of intervention on the primary endpoint of interest is reliably predicted using the surrogate endpoint. Fleming and DeMets (1996) provide several examples where misleading results have been obtained using surrogate endpoints, indicating how difficult it is to obtain such reliable predictions in practice.
7. Investigators might consider adopting a stratified or matched-pair design, recognizing that it is only worthwhile to match or stratify on baseline variables which are strongly related to outcome, and further taking into account the analytic limitations associated with pair-matching (see Section 3.6). Adjustment in the statistical analysis for other baseline variables associated with the study outcome can also lead to improved power.

8. Some gain in power may be obtained by taking repeated assessments over time from the same subjects or from different samples of subjects. For example, the REACT trial described in Section 5.2.2 adopted such a strategy (Feldman *et al.* 1998). The primary design for this trial involved 10 matched pairs of communities, in which a randomly selected member of each pair received an educational campaign aimed at reducing treatment-seeking delay for the acute symptoms of myocardial infarction. Recognizing that the number of matched pairs was small, the investigators attempted to improve the power of the trial by taking repeated measurements on the same communities over time. The primary response variable at the community level was then defined as the slope of the linear trend of mean log delay time as computed over the course of the repeated measures.

   In general, the gain in efficiency obtained through the use of repeated measurements in cluster randomization trials must be always balanced against the added cost and administrative complexity that will be involved.

# 6

# Analysis of binary outcomes

Methods for analysing binary (dichotomous) outcome data in cluster randomization trials are not as well established as methods for analysing continuous outcome data (discussed in Ch. 7). As a consequence, many researchers have either treated binary outcome data as continuous in their analyses or completely ignored the clustering for such outcomes. The analytic issues involved are complicated by the absence of a unique multivariate extension of the binomial distribution analogous to the multivariate normal distribution, and by the fact that there is no single approach that has uniformly superior properties. Thus the investigator must deal with a bewildering array of possible approaches to the data analysis. This is true even for the simplest designs, in which clusters of fixed size are randomized to each of several intervention groups, and without considering the need for baseline covariate adjustment, at either the cluster or the individual level. Moreover, most of the available methods require a fairly large number of clusters per intervention group in order to assure their validity.

The simplest approach to analysing binary data from a cluster randomization trial is to obtain a single summary score for each cluster. Then the analysis can be conducted at the same level as the random assignment using standard statistical procedures. In Section 6.1 we review the advantages and disadvantages of this strategy, noting in particular its connections to more technically sophisticated individual-level analyses.

A well-established principle in scientific experimentation is that the analytic approach adopted should correspond to the underlying design. Although many cluster randomization trials have ignored this principle, e.g. by not taking into account design-based stratification or matching, this practice cannot be routinely encouraged, since, in general, it leads to loss of power if the stratification is effective. Methods specifically suited to the completely randomized design, the matched-pair design and the stratified design are therefore described in Sections 6.2, 6.3 and 6.4, respectively.

Although most randomized trials are designed under the assumption that the units allocated are of equal size, this assumption will usually not be tenable at the analysis stage. For example, virtually all prospective studies experience some loss to follow-up of subjects, and this is likely to occur disproportionately among the allocated clusters. Even in cross-sectional studies involving 'natural' units such as schools or medical practices, some variation in cluster size can be expected unless a deliberate subsampling scheme is adopted. Thus in Chapters 6–8, we will assume, unless otherwise stated, that the required statistical analysis will involve clusters of unequal size. The numbers of clusters per intervention group may also be unequal, on either a planned or an unplanned basis.

## 6.1 Selecting the unit of analysis

Although we focus specifically in this chapter on the analysis of binary outcome data, much of the discussion in this section remains relevant for any selected outcome variable. The key issues are summarized in Table 6.1.

A point we have made repeatedly is that the unit of inference in cluster randomization trials may be directed either at the cluster level or at the level of the individual subject. In many trials, an interest in cluster-level inferences leads investigators to collect data only at the cluster level. For example, in Section 3.3 we described how one of the secondary aims of the Child and Adolescent Trial for Cardiovascular Health (CATCH) was to assess the effect of training food service personnel on how to improve the dietary content of lunch menus. The resulting analysis of dietary content was then naturally conducted at the cluster (school) level. Thus the challenge in selecting a unit of analysis is particularly acute when data are available from individual study subjects. Nevertheless, such data are often available regardless of the unit of inference. This may reflect investigator uncertainty regarding what is the most appropriate level of inference or, alternatively, may simply reflect the fact that data are more naturally and easily obtained at the individual level.

The investigator faced with analysing individual-level data must account for the lack of statistical independence among observations within a cluster. A method of

**Table 6.1** Comparing cluster-level and individual-level analyses

*Advantages of cluster-level analyses*
- Easy to conduct and explain
- Can be applied to any outcome variable
- Permit the construction of exact statistical inferences
- Can be adapted to adjust for baseline imbalance and/or variability in cluster size
- When properly weighted will provide power comparable to individual-level analyses

*Advantages of individual-level analyses*
- Reduce to standard statistical procedures in the absence of clustering
- Allow more direct examination of the joint effects of cluster-level and individual-level predictors
- Can be extended to permit analyses of multilevel data
- More naturally yield estimates of intracluster correlation coefficients
- Will provide more efficient estimates of the effect of intervention than unweighted analyses when there are many clusters per group, particularly when cluster sizes are highly variable

simplifying the problem is to collapse the data in each cluster, followed by the construction of a meaningful summary measure, such as an average, to serve as the unit of analysis. Standard statistical methods can then be directly applied to the collapsed measures. This removes the problem of non-independence since the subsequent significance tests and confidence intervals would be based on the variation among cluster summary values rather than on the variation among individuals.

Cluster-level analyses can also be used for more complex summary scores (e.g. trend over time) and, more generally, for any study outcome. The choice of an appropriate summary score in a given trial will depend on the primary question of interest. However, any such decision should be clearly specified in advance of the data collection, and ideally noted in the study protocol. This helps to protect investigators against claims that a summary score was selected because it maximized the difference across intervention groups, and also helps to focus the problem of determining sample size (Koepsell *et al.* 1991).

Cluster-level analyses are most obviously appropriate when the primary questions of interest focus more on the randomized unit as a whole than on the individual subjects, since this becomes the most direct way of addressing the study aims. An example of this approach is provided by Oakeshott *et al.* (1994), who describe a trial in which the primary endpoint was the percentage of X-ray examinations requested by a general practitioner that met certain guidelines. In this study, previously discussed in Section 1.5, the responses of individual practice patients were not of direct interest.

Questions concerning the appropriate unit of analysis are more challenging when the primary target of inference is at the level of the individual subject, with the choice of randomization unit then largely a matter of convenience or other practical considerations. For example, in the birth attendant trial described in Chapter 1 (Bullough *et al.* 1989), it was the individual mother at whom the intervention was directly aimed and who was the main focus of interest. Birth attendants were chosen as the unit of randomization solely for logistical reasons and to avoid the likelihood of treatment contamination. Similarly, in the hypertension screening and management trial, also described in Chapter 1 (Bass *et al.*1986), outcomes on an individual patient level were of prime interest, with practical considerations alone dictating the decision to randomize intact practices.

Particular care must be taken when conducting individual-level analyses to properly adjust for the effects of clustering. A variety of different approaches are available. For example, in Section 6.2 we describe how estimates of the intracluster correlation coefficient may be used to calculate a variance inflation factor adjusting the Pearson chi-square test for the effect of clustering. For most approaches, the validity of individual-level analyses requires a relatively large number of clusters per intervention group. Unfortunately, the alternative strategy of sampling a large number of subjects per cluster is not sufficient to ensure the validity of these analyses. However, exact statistical inferences for cluster-level analyses can be constructed based on the randomization (permutation) distribution for the selected summary statistic. These inferences will be valid in samples of any size, although often lacking in power.

An important special case arises in trials having a quantitative outcome variable when each cluster has a fixed number of subjects. In this case, exact statistical inferences concerning the effect of intervention can be constructed using standard analysis of variance. Moreover, the resulting test statistic is algebraically identical to the test statistic obtained using a cluster-level analysis (Hopkins 1982, Koepsell *et al.* 1991). The implication from this identity is that for quantitative outcome variables, a cluster-level analysis is fully efficient when all clusters are of the same size. Thus the suggestion which is sometimes made that a cluster-level analysis intrinsically assumes $\rho = 1$ is misleading, since such an analysis can be efficiently conducted regardless of the value of $\rho$. It is important to note, however, that this equivalence between cluster-level and individual-level analyses, which holds exactly for quantitative outcome variables under balance, holds only approximately for binary outcome variables.

In practice, the number of subjects per cluster will tend to exhibit considerable variability, either by design or by subject attrition. Cluster-level analyses which give equal weight to all clusters may then prove to be imprecise. This suggests that weighted cluster-level analyses should then be conducted to account for such variability (e.g. Bland and Kerry 1998, Marubini *et al.* 1988). Standard statistical theory shows that the precision of these analyses is maximized when the cluster-level summary score is weighted inversely proportional to the reciprocal of its estimated variance. This implies that the optimal weights are usually a function of both the cluster sizes and the degree of intracluster correlation. If there are only a small number of clusters per intervention group, however, imprecision in the estimation of these weights might result in a loss of power (e.g. Shao, 1990) relative to an unweighted analysis. Thus, in practice, large gains in power due to weighting are not assured. Furthermore, when there are a large number of clusters, appropriately weighted cluster-level analyses are again equivalent to individual-level analyses (Marubini *et al.* 1988, Raudenbush 1993).

Some potential gain in power for testing the effect of intervention may also be obtained by adjusting for imbalances in baseline predictors of study outcome. Individual-level analyses conducted using regression models may then prove preferable, since they can be used to examine the joint effects of both cluster-level (e.g. percentage of smokers) and individual-level predictors (e.g. individual smoking status) on outcome (Hedeker *et al.* 1994a, Kreft 1998). Estimates of intracluster correlation coefficients are also more naturally obtained as part of an individual-level analysis (e.g. Murray and Short 1997).

A variety of methods have been developed to adjust cluster-level analyses for imbalances in baseline predictors across intervention groups. For example, direct standardization can be used to obtain cluster-specific summary scores adjusted for specified baseline variables (Smith and Morrow 1991, pp. 307–309). Similar strategies have been used in a variety of cluster randomization trials (e.g. Bass *et al.* 1986, Gail *et al.* 1996) and should be considered if only as part of a sensitivity analysis when there are too few clusters to support the more stringent assumptions of a model-based individual-level analysis. Note that standard multiple regression methods applied at the cluster level are sufficient to adjust for baseline imbalance on those predictors which are also measured at that level, e.g. cluster size and geographic location.

Concern for the ecological fallacy (Morgenstern 1998) has been raised as an argument against the use of cluster-level analyses (e.g. Kreft 1998). Such concerns may be misplaced. The primary analysis of the effect of intervention in most randomized trials includes all eligible subjects regardless of their compliance with the protocol. This strategy, known as 'analysis by intention-to-treat' (Pocock 1983, pp. 182–186, Piantadosi 1997, pp. 276–281), is particularly attractive because it is the only analysis protected by random assignment. The ecological fallacy cannot arise in this case since the assigned intervention is shared by all cluster members.

Intention-to-treat analyses may be conducted using either the individual or the cluster as the unit of analysis. As with any intent-to-treat analysis, however, inferences are most appropriately interpreted as evaluating the effect of instituting a treatment policy (e.g. a smoking cessation programme). Nonetheless, investigators are also often interested in evaluating the effect of intervention as administered and received according to the protocol. These 'efficacy analyses' therefore require some measurement of the degree to which the intervention was actually received by a given subject. For example, reports of students' attendance might be used as a proxy measure of the degree to which a smoking prevention programme was received in school-based cluster randomization trials. The subsequent analyses of fully compliant students could again be conducted at either the individual or the cluster level, although the interpretation of such subgroup analyses is no longer protected by random assignment.

The remarks above do not imply that the ecological fallacy should be ignored in all analyses. Consider CATCH, a school-based trial for cardiovascular health (Luepker *et al.* 1996). One of the trial outcomes for this study was body mass index. The effect of intervention on this outcome might well vary depending on both a child's obesity at the start of the trial relative to other students from the same school and the average degree of obesity at the school level. Individual-level analyses conducted using multilevel (hierarchical) models (e.g. Duncan *et al.* 1998) most easily permit examination of these possibly distinct effects of intervention. The ecological fallacy could result if heterogeneity in the effect of intervention found at the school level was wrongly taken to imply heterogeneity at the level of the individual student. There is, of course, only very limited power for conducting such secondary analyses. Moreover, while these analyses may enrich our understanding of the trial results, they are almost always exploratory in nature.

The selection of an appropriate unit of analysis can be fairly complicated in some trials. Consider, for example, the Television School and Family Smoking Prevention and Cessation Project described by Hedeker *et al.* (1994a). Participating schools were randomly assigned to one of four intervention groups in a $2 \times 2$ factorial design. Analyses could be carried out at the student, classroom or school level. However, analyses conducted at either the student or classroom level need to account for the correlation between responses of students from the same school, since schools were the unit of randomization.

Challenges in identifying and distinguishing the unit of inference, the unit of analysis and the impact of clustering are not unique to cluster randomization trials. Indeed, many of the ideas presented in this section are based on earlier discussions of methods for the analysis of longitudinal or repeated-measures data (Matthews *et al.* 1990). Related discussions have also taken place among epidemiologists (von Korff *et al.* 1992), nursing researchers (Gilliss and Davis 1992) and in studies of primary care (Whiting-O'Keefe *et al.* 1984). Data arising from primary care studies, for example, may be analysed at the patient level, family level, health care provider level or practice level. Thus the resulting analyses can be more complicated than is typically the case for randomized trials, in which the effect of clustering is induced by the unit of randomization. It follows that decisions regarding the unit of analysis and the impact of clustering depend much more on subject matter expertise when clustering is not a consequence of study design. This is the case for cluster randomization trials as well as for complex surveys using cluster sampling.

## 6.2 The completely randomized design

### 6.2.1 Comparison of proportions

The principal aim of many cluster randomization designs is to compare the proportion of individuals in different intervention groups who have a specified characteristic, such as the development of disease by a fixed point in time. For the sake of simplicity, we will focus on the most frequently occurring case of a two-group intervention study, although all the procedures discussed can be generalized in a natural way to allow the comparison of more than two groups. Suppose that $k_i$ clusters are randomized to intervention group $i$ $(i = 1, 2)$, with $m_{ij}$ denoting the size of the $j$th cluster in group $i$, and $Y_{ijl}$, $l = 1, \ldots, m_{ij}$ denoting the binary outcome for the $l$th subject from the $ij$th cluster. Then for subjects with the outcome of interest (e.g. development of disease), we let $Y_{ijl} = 1$ and otherwise let $Y_{ijl} = 0$. Then $Y_{ij} = \sum_{l=1}^{m_{ij}} Y_{ijl}$ denotes the corresponding number of subjects with disease (i.e. number of successes), and $\hat{P}_{ij} = Y_{ij}/m_{ij}$ denotes the cluster-specific event rate, $j = 1, 2, \ldots, k_i$. Group 1, for example, may correspond to an educational intervention as applied to a sample of $k_1$ clusters, while group 2 may correspond to a control intervention as applied to $k_2$ clusters. The rates $\hat{P}_{ij}$ denote the proportion of subjects in a cluster who develop the specified characteristic over the length of the study. It is also convenient to define the following notation:

$Y_i = \sum_{j=1}^{k_i} Y_{ij}$ = total number of successes in group $i$

$M_i = \sum_{j=1}^{k_i} m_{ij}$ = total number of individuals in group $i$

$K = \sum_{i=1}^{2} k_i$ = total number of clusters in the study

$M = \sum_{i=1}^{2} M_i$ = total number of individuals in the study

$Y = \sum_{i=1}^{2} Y_i$ = total number of successes in the study

$\hat{P}_i = \sum_{j=1}^{k_i} Y_{ij} / \sum_{j=1}^{k_i} m_{ij} = Y_i/M_i$ = event rate as computed over all clusters in group $i$

$\hat{P} = \sum_{i=1}^{2} Y_i / \sum_{i=1}^{2} M_i = Y/M$ = overall event rate observed in the study.

Assuming a common value for the intracluster correlation coefficient $\rho$, a pooled estimate of this parameter is obtained by applying the standard analysis of variance formula to the (0,1) binary observations, where 0 denotes a failure and 1 a success.

Letting

$$\bar{m}_{Ai} = \sum_{j=1}^{k_i} m_{ij}^2 / M_i$$

the resulting estimator of $\rho$ may be written as

$$\hat{\rho} = \frac{\text{MSC} - \text{MSW}}{\text{MSC} + (m_0 - 1)\text{MSW}}$$

where

$$\text{MSC} = \sum_{i=1}^{2} \sum_{j=1}^{k_i} m_{ij}(\hat{P}_{ij} - \hat{P}_i)^2 / (K - 2)$$

$$\text{MSW} = \sum_{i=1}^{2} \sum_{j=1}^{k_i} m_{ij}\hat{P}_{ij}(1 - \hat{P}_{ij}) / (M - K)$$

and

$$m_0 = \left[ M - \sum_{i=1}^{2} \bar{m}_{Ai} \right] / (K - 2)$$

and where MSC and MSW are the pooled mean square errors between and within clusters, respectively.

Note that if responses on subjects within a cluster are no more similar than responses on subjects in different clusters, then MSC = MSW and $\hat{\rho} = 0$. If all responses within a cluster are identically equal to zero or one, then MSW = 0 and $\hat{\rho} - 1$. Negative values of $\hat{\rho}$ are usually taken to indicate sampling error, and thus set equal to zero.

There are a number of procedures that may be used to test $H_0$: $P_1 = P_2$, which we now review in detail. To make ideas concrete, the discussion below will take place in the context of a particular example. The example involves data obtained from a study evaluating the effect of school-based interventions in reducing adolescent tobacco use (Murray *et al.* 1992), and previously considered by Donner and Klar (1994b). In this study, 12 schools were randomly assigned to each of four conditions, including three experimental conditions and a control condition (existing curriculum). For each school, the number of students engaged in different types of smoking behaviour was recorded at various follow-up times. For the purposes of illustration, we are interested here in comparing the effect of the Smoke Free Generation intervention with the existing curriculum on the proportion of children who report using smokeless tobacco after 2 years of follow-up. The data for this comparison are presented in Table 6.2, where it is seen that the overall observed rates of tobacco use in the experimental and control groups are 0.043 and 0.062, respectively. In the following sections we discuss several approaches that may be taken to test the hypothesis that the true event rates are equal, beginning with one approach that is best referred to as 'naive'.

#### *6.2.1.1 Standard Pearson chi-square test*

As noted in Chapter 1, investigators frequently use inappropriate methods, such as the Pearson chi-square statistic, to test the effect of intervention in cluster randomization

**Table 6.2:** Proportion of children who report using smokeless tobacco after 2 years of follow-up in each of 12 schools randomly assigned to one of two conditions (Murray *et al.* 1992)

| Smoke Free Generation[a] | Existing Curriculum[a] |
|---|---|
| 0/42 | 5/103 |
| 1/84 | 3/174 |
| 9/149 | 6/83 |
| 11/136 | 6/75 |
| 4/58 | 2/152 |
| 1/55 | 7/102 |
| 10/219 | 7/104 |
| 4/160 | 3/74 |
| 2/63 | 1/55 |
| 5/85 | 23/225 |
| 1/96 | 16/125 |
| 10/194 | 12/207 |

[a] Overall rates of tobacco use: Smoke Free Generation, 58/1341 = 0.043; Existing Curriculum, 91/1479 = 0.062.

trials. Application of this statistic to comparing the overall event rates in the two groups yields

$$\chi^2_P = \sum_{i=1}^{2} \frac{M_i(\hat{P}_i - \hat{P})^2}{\hat{P}(1-\hat{P})}$$

$$= \frac{1341(0.043-0.053)^2}{0.053(1-0.053)} + \frac{1479(0.062-0.053)^2}{0.053(1-0.053)}$$

$$= 4.69 \quad (p = 0.03)$$

This result might be taken to imply that the use of smokeless tobacco among experimental group individuals is significantly reduced as compared with control group individuals. However, a fundamental assumption of this procedure is that the sample observations are statistically independent. This assumption is almost certainly violated here, since it is more reasonable to assume that responses taken on subjects within a school are more similar than responses taken on subjects in different schools, i.e. to assume that the intracluster correlation coefficient $\rho$ is positive. This would imply that the computed $p$-value of 0.03 is likely to be biased downward and that the difference in observed event rates may not in fact be statistically significant at the 5 per cent level. The magnitude of the bias associated with $\chi^2_P$ increases with both the value of $\rho$ and the average cluster size. For clusters of fixed size $m$, the bias is given by the variance inflation factor $[1 + (m-1)\rho]$. Thus, for example, if $\rho = 0.01$ and $m = 100$, the value of $\chi^2_P$ will tend to be spuriously inflated by a factor of approximately 2.0.

A similar concern applies to other standard procedures for comparing proportions, such as Fisher's exact test (Armitage and Berry 1994). The validity of this procedure also depends on the assumption of statistical independence among the sample observations.

Inappropriate application of these procedures to clustered data is sometimes referred to as the 'unit of analysis error'. However, this terminology is misleading, as it confuses the choice of analytic unit with the need to account for the impact of clustering, issues which are conceptually quite different.

#### 6.2.1.2 Cluster-level analyses

**Two-sample $t$-test comparing average values of the event rates**

Researchers who have recognized the pitfalls involved in applying $\chi^2_P$ to clustered data have adopted a variety of alternative procedures. One common approach has been to test whether the difference between the average values of the event rates in the two groups is statistically significant using the standard two-sample (unpaired) $t$-test. The unweighted mean event rates may be computed as $\overline{P}_1$ and $\overline{P}_2$ for the experimental and control groups respectively, where

$$\overline{P}_i = \sum_{j=1}^{k_i} \hat{P}_{ij}/k_i \qquad i = 1, 2$$

We denote the sample variances of the observed event rates in the two groups by $S_1^2$ and $S_2^2$, respectively, where

$$S_i^2 = \sum_{j=1}^{k_i} (\hat{P}_{ij} - \overline{P}_i)^2/(k_i - 1) \qquad i = 1, 2$$

Then the two sample unpaired $t$-statistic is given by

$$t_u = (\overline{P}_1 - \overline{P}_2) \Big/ \sqrt{S^2\left(\frac{1}{k_1} + \frac{1}{k_2}\right)}$$

where $S^2 = \{(k_1 - 1)S_1^2 + (k_2 - 1)S_2^2\}/(K - 2)$ is the pooled error variance. For the data in Table 6.2, we have $\overline{P}_1 - \overline{P}_2 = 0.039 - 0.060 = -0.021$ and $S^2 = 11[0.026^2 + 0.035^2]/22 = 0.000\,95$. Under the null hypothesis of no difference between the true mean event rates, $t_u$ follows an approximate $t$-distribution with $K - 2$ degrees of freedom. The resulting value of the test statistic with 22 degrees of freedom is then given by

$$t_u = (-0.021) \Big/ \sqrt{0.000\,95\left(\frac{2}{12}\right)} = -1.67 \quad (p = 0.11)$$

A theoretical objection that may be raised against this approach is that the assumptions required for the validity of the $t$-test are not strictly satisfied. These assumptions are essentially that the cluster-specific event rates are normally distributed with equal variances. Clearly, these assumptions are violated here, particularly if there is considerable variation in cluster size. Nevertheless, extensive simulation research has shown that the $t$-test is remarkably robust to violations of the underlying assumptions (e.g. Heeren and D'Agostino 1987, Donner and Klar 1996), particularly when there are equal numbers of clusters assigned to each intervention group. A related objection that may be raised to the use of this procedure is that it completely ignores any variation in cluster size, placing each of the observed event rates on the same footing. Assuming there are enough clusters to ensure that $\rho$ is accurately estimated, potentially improved power may be obtained using weights proportional to the reciprocal of $\text{Var}(\hat{P}_{ij})$, given by $W_{ij} = m_{ij}/[1 + (m_{ij} - 1)\rho]$. Moreover, when all clusters are of large size, $W_{ij} \simeq 1/\rho$ does not depend on the values of the $m_{ij}$, so that unweighted analyses will tend to be as fully efficient as weighted analyses. An alternative strategy is to transform the observed proportions to a scale on which the required assumptions are more closely adhered to, e.g. the arcsine scale.

**Non-parametric approaches**

The strict lack of applicability of the parametric $t$-test suggests that a non-parametric approach which makes no assumptions about the distribution of the school-specific event rates may be preferable for testing the effect of intervention. A natural approach here is the Wilcoxon rank sum test, a non-parametric procedure based on the ranks of observed event rates. This procedure, also known as the Mann–Whitney $U$-test, requires that the two groups be pooled and the event rates ranked by size. The underlying rationale is that if the intervention has no effect, the sum of the ranks for each group should be the same. Let $T_i$ $(i = 1, 2)$, denote the sum of the ranks for the $i$th group. Provided that there are at least 15 clusters per intervention group (i.e. $k_i \geqslant 15$, $i = 1, 2$) the test is performed by referring

$$Z_W = \frac{T_1 - \dfrac{k_1(k_1 + k_2 + 1)}{2}}{\sqrt{k_1 k_2(k_1 + k_2 + 1)/12}}$$

to tables of the standard normal distribution. Investigators applying this test who are faced with an excessive number of tied observations could apply one of the suggested corrections for improving the normal approximation in this case (e.g. Conover 1980, p. 217, Rosner 1995, Section 12.4).

The number of schools per group in this example is fairly small ($k_1 = k_2 = 12$), suggesting that an exact test may be preferable. Moreover, the observed event rates for two of the schools are identical, implying that the validity of the normal approximation becomes even more questionable. Based on the usual strategy of assigning the mean rank for tied event rates, we have $T_1 = 125.5$, $T_2 = 174.5$ and

$$Z_W = \frac{125.5 - \dfrac{12(24 + 1)}{2}}{\sqrt{(12)(12)(24 + 1)/12}}$$
$$= -1.41 \quad (p = 0.16)$$

Since the number of clusters in each group is fairly small, it may be preferable to compute an exact $p$-value for these data, particularly since standard tables (e.g. Rosner 1995, Table 13) strictly apply only in the absence of tied event rates. The exact test may be readily calculated using software packages such as Proc-StatXact (Mehta and Patel, 1997), which for these data again gives a $p$-value of 0.16. This result may be interpreted as a failure to reject the hypothesis that the rates of tobacco use are different among schools assigned to the two conditions.

There is no question as to the validity of applying non-parametric methods to the ranks of the original observations. However, it is a validity gained at the expense of precision, i.e. a reduced ability to detect important intervention effects. This is because inference procedures based on ranks ignore not only variations in cluster size, but also the actual magnitudes of the event rates. This loss of information is reflected by the fact that unless the number of clusters per group is at least four, it is impossible to achieve two-sided statistical significance at $p < 0.05$, regardless of the magnitude of the intervention effect.

An alternative non-parametric approach that does take into account the values of the cluster-specific event rates is Fisher's two-sample permutation test (Conover 1980, Section 5.11). This procedure is based on considering the number of different ways in which the cluster-specific event rates could be permuted (randomized) between intervention groups while maintaining the same number of clusters per group. No other distributional or model-based assumptions are made. An appropriately selected test statistic (e.g. the difference in mean event rates for data in Table 6.2) is then calculated for each such permutation. The two-sided statistical significance of the test is equal to the proportion of test statistics found using the permuted data that are at least as large, in absolute value, as the test statistic found using the observed data. As is the case with the Wilcoxon rank sum test, which is simply the permutation test based on ranks, at least four clusters per group are needed in a two-group comparison to obtain two-sided statistical significance at $p < 0.05$.

An approximate version of the permutation test may be obtained by computing the standard error of the difference in mean event rates under the randomization procedure discussed above. Under the null hypothesis of no intervention effect, the estimated standard error of $\overline{P}_1 - \overline{P}_2$ is given by

$$\widehat{\mathrm{SE}}(P_1 - P_2) = \left\{ \frac{\sum_{i=1}^{2} \sum_{j=1}^{k_i} (\hat{P}_{ij} - \overline{P})^2}{K - 1} \left( \frac{1}{k_1} + \frac{1}{k_2} \right) \right\}^{1/2}$$

where

$$\bar{P} = \sum_{i=1}^{2} \sum_{j=1}^{k_i} \hat{P}_{ij} / K$$

For the data in Table 6.2, an approximate normal deviate test statistic may then be computed as

$$\begin{aligned} Z_{\mathrm{PT}} &= (\overline{P}_1 - \overline{P}_2) / \widehat{\mathrm{SE}}(\overline{P}_1 - \overline{P}_2) \\ &= -0.021/0.013 = -1.61 \quad (p = 0.11) \end{aligned}$$

Using the package Proc-StatXact (Mehta and Patel 1997), an exact $p$-value for the two-sample permutation test is given by 0.11. This package may also be used to obtain exact $p$-values for permutation tests involving more than two groups, although the computational demands are considerably increased.

Gail *et al.* (1996) have studied the properties of permutation tests as applied to both completely randomized and matched-pair cluster randomization designs. They also show how interval estimates of intervention effects based on permutation tests may be obtained. However, the individual-level analyses described in the following section might prove more practical since they more naturally lend themselves to inferences on the odds ratio scale. This scale is frequently the most preferred in practice for analysing dichotomous data, particularly when multivariate analyses are also conducted.

### 6.2.1.3 Individual-level analyses

The analyses discussed in Section 6.2.1.2, based on the application of the $t$-test or its non-parametric analogues, are all performed at the cluster level. We now describe several alternative approaches that may be conducted at the level of the individual subject. One individual-level approach for testing the difference between event rates is to empirically adjust the standard chi-square test for the clustering of responses within a randomized unit. This relatively simple method is intuitively attractive since it yields the standard Pearson chi-square statistic if the estimated intracluster coefficient $\hat{\rho}$ is zero, and is easily extended to the comparison of more than two groups. It also imposes no distributional assumptions on the responses within a cluster.

**Adjusted chi-square approach**

Donner and Donald (1988) proposed an adjustment that depends on computing clustering correction factors for each group given by

$$C_i = \left\{ \sum_{j=1}^{k_i} m_{ij}[1 + (m_{ij} - 1)\hat{\rho}] \right\} \Big/ \sum_{j=1}^{k_i} m_{ij} = 1 + (\overline{m}_{Ai} - 1)\hat{\rho} \qquad i = 1, 2$$

The factor $C_i$ can be thought of as the estimated or observed design effect in group $i$, where the population design effect measures the inflation in variance of $\hat{P}_i$ that can be attributed to clustering. An assumption behind this adjustment approach is that $C_1$ and $C_2$ estimate the same population design effect, i.e. are not significantly different. This assumption is guaranteed to hold (at least under $H_0$) for experimental comparisons, but may not hold for non-randomized comparisons in which clusters are systematically assigned to receive different interventions.

For the data in Table 6.2, we have $\hat{\rho} = 0.01$, with $C_1 = 2.536$ and $C_2 = 2.599$. The values of the estimated design effects indicate that the variance of the observed event rates in each group has more than doubled as a result of the clustering of responses within schools. They also show that even a small value of $\hat{\rho}$, combined with a fairly large average cluster size, can lead to a very substantial design effect.

The adjusted one degree of freedom chi-square statistic is then given by

$$\begin{aligned} \chi^2_A &= \sum_{i=1}^{2} \frac{M_i(\hat{P}_i - \hat{P})^2}{C_i\hat{P}(1 - \hat{P})} \\ &= \frac{1341(0.043 - 0.053)^2}{2.536(0.053)(1 - 0.053)} + \frac{1479(0.062 - 0.053)^2}{2.599(0.053)(1 - 0.053)} \\ &= 1.83 \quad (p = 0.18) \end{aligned}$$

Note that while the value of the unadjusted chi-square statistic was clearly significant at the five per cent level, $\chi^2_A$ is not statistically significant at any conventional level.

Klar *et al.* (1995) used this procedure to compare parasitic infection rates in a tropical medicine field trial randomizing families to different screening and treatment programmes (see Gyorkos *et al.* 1989). A further example in the context of data arising from ophthalmological studies is given by Donner (1989).

It is important to note that the validity of the adjusted chi-square test statistic does not depend on the assumption that the pairwise correlation between any two observations in the same cluster is constant, i.e. it does not require an 'exchangeable' correlation structure. In the case of a heterogeneous correlation structure, $\hat{\rho}$ measures the average degree of pairwise correlation (assumed to be constant across clusters), and the statistic $\chi_A^2$ remains valid (Klar 1996). If the true within-cluster correlation structure were known, adjustments to the Pearson chi-square statistic could be developed that, in theory, would be more efficient. However, such detailed prior information will only rarely be available. An example of the adjusted chi-square test as extended to the comparison of more than two event rates is provided by Donner and Donald (1988).

**Ratio estimator approach**

This approach, like the one described in the previous section, is also based on a relatively simple adjustment of the standard Pearson chi-square statistic. However, the concept of design effect, based on regarding the event rate $\hat{P}_i = Y_i/M_i$ as a ratio rather than as a proportion, is developed quite differently. If individuals rather than clusters were the unit of allocation, then the estimated variance of $\hat{P}_i$ would be given by the usual binomial expression $\widehat{\text{Var}}_B(\hat{P}_i) = \hat{P}_i(1 - \hat{P}_i)/M_i$. However, $\widehat{\text{Var}}_B(\hat{P}_i)$ tends to underestimate the true variance of $\hat{P}_i$ if the unit of allocation is an intact cluster. Technically we say that $\hat{P}_i$ is overdispersed relative to a binomial random variable. If $\hat{P}_i$ is regarded as a ratio, an appropriate variance estimate is obtained from standard sample survey theory (Cochran 1977) as

$$\widehat{\text{Var}}_R(\hat{P}_i) = k_i(k_i - 1)^{-1} M_i^{-2} \sum_{j-1}^{k_i} (Y_{ij} - m_{ij}\hat{P}_i)^2$$

The estimated design effect in group $i$ is then defined as $d_i = \widehat{\text{Var}}_R(\hat{P}_i)/\widehat{\text{Var}}_B(\hat{P}_i)$. For the data in Table 6.2, the estimated design effects are given by $d_1 = 1.39$ and $d_2 = 3.58$, respectively.

The estimates $d_i$ may be used directly to adjust the standard Pearson chi-square statistic for the effect of clustering. Let $\widetilde{M}_i = M_i/d_i$, $\widetilde{Y}_i = Y_i/d_i$ and

$$\widetilde{P} = \sum_{i=1}^{2} \widetilde{Y}_i \bigg/ \sum_{i=1}^{2} \widetilde{M}_i$$

Then the one degree of freedom ratio estimator chi-square statistic (Rao and Scott 1992) is given by

$$\chi_R^2 = \sum_{i=1}^{2} \frac{\widetilde{M}_i(\hat{P}_i - \widetilde{P})^2}{\widetilde{P}(1 - \widetilde{P})}$$

Note that this statistic is identical to $\chi_P^2$, with the adjusted sample estimates $\widetilde{M}_i$ and $\widetilde{P}$ replacing $M_i$ and $\hat{P}$, respectively. Thus, operationally, the ratio estimator approach simply involves dividing the observed counts in the Pearson chi-square statistic by an estimate of the design effect, hence reducing the effective sample size. However, unlike the statistic $\chi_A^2$ described in this section, the statistic $\chi_R^2$ does not, in general, reduce to $\chi_P^2$ if the intracluster correlation is estimated as zero. In fact, this procedure does not explicitly involve the notion of an intracluster correlation at all.

For the data in Table 6.2, we have

$$\chi^2_R = \frac{1341(0.043 - 0.049)^2}{1.39(0.049)(1 - 0.049)} + \frac{1479(0.062 - 0.049)^2}{3.58(0.049)(1 - 0.049)}$$
$$= 2.08 \quad (p = 0.15)$$

The ratio estimator approach does not require the assumption that the population design effects in the two comparison groups are equal. Thus it is well suited to non-randomized comparisons, particularly those involving systematic differences in mean cluster size from group to group. However, for trials involving the random allocation of clusters to different intervention groups, the assumption of a common design effect is guaranteed, at least under $H_0$. Hence the statistic $\chi^2_A$ is generally more appropriate than $\chi^2_R$ for randomized comparisons. Evidence also suggests (e.g. Donner *et al.* 1994) that the number of clusters per group required to ensure the validity of $\chi^2_R$ may be fairly substantial (at least 20 per group). From a statistical perspective, the statistic $\chi^2_R$ performs best under conditions which ensure the optimal performance of the ratio estimator as recommended for its use in sample survey research: a large number of clusters and a relatively small degree of variation in cluster size (Cochran 1977, Ch. 6). Note, however, that Fung *et al.* (1994) discussed various modifications of the statistic $\chi^2_R$ that may improve its performance in small to moderate-sized samples.

**Parametric modelling**

This approach is fully parametric in the sense that the subject responses are assumed to follow a specified probability distribution. One choice is the beta-binomial distribution, which results when (i) the number of responses within a cluster follows a binomial distribution conditional on the probability parameter $P_{ij}$, and (ii) the cluster-specific success rates $P_{ij}$ are assumed to vary across clusters in accordance with a beta distribution. The latter assumption implies that the resulting beta-binomial distribution will exhibit more variability than the binomial distribution but will essentially reduce to the latter when the intracluster correlation coefficient $\rho$ is zero. In this sense we say that the beta-binomial distribution is 'overdispersed' relative to the binomial distribution.

The parameters of the beta-binomial distribution may be estimated using the method of maximum likelihood, which leads to a likelihood ratio test of the null hypothesis that a single beta-binomial distribution can be used to fit the observations. Interestingly, this test assumes a common value of the intracluster correlation $\rho$ in each group, but not necessarily a common design effect. Compared with the methods previously described, it is also computationally intensive, requiring an iterative solution using numerical maximization techniques. For the data in Table 6.2, the resulting chi-square statistic, with one degree of freedom, is given by $\chi^2_B = 1.81$ $(p = 0.18)$. A two degree of freedom likelihood ratio test may also be developed in which the assumption of a common $\rho$ is relaxed (Williams 1975). Such a test would be sensitive to the effect of intervention on either the underlying event rate or the value of the intracluster correlation, a test which is usually of less direct interest to investigators than one which focuses specifically on the difference in event rates.

Likelihood ratio procedures based on other parametric distributions may also be developed for testing the equality of event rates in cluster randomization trials.

These include the logistic-normal likelihood ratio test (Neuhaus 1992) and the probit-normal likelihood ratio test (Hedeker *et al.* 1994a). They differ from the beta-binomial likelihood ratio test with respect to the specific assumptions made regarding the nature of the between-cluster variability. The first of these procedures assumes that the logit transform of the $P_{ij}$ follows a normal distribution across clusters, while the second imposes a similar assumption on the probit transform of the $P_{ij}$. One advantage of the logistic-normal and probit-normal models is that they can be readily extended to model dependence on individual-level covariates. For the data in Table 6.2, the one degree of freedom likelihood ratio chi-square statistic from the logistic-normal model is given by $\chi^2_{LN} = 1.97$ ($p = 0.16$). A weakness of both the logistic-normal and the probit-normal models is that the resulting estimates of intervention effect may not be simple to interpret (see Neuhaus 1992).

Likelihood ratio tests based on the logistic-normal or the beta-binomial distributions can be constructed using the software package EGRET (1990), where these procedures are provided as extensions of standard logistic regression models. These tests may also be obtained by using MIXOR, a computer program for mixed effects ordinal regression models (Hedeker and Gibbons 1996), or MlwiN, a software package developed by the Multilevel Models Project (Goldstein *et al.* 1998). Inferences based on the closely related mixed effects logistic regression models are available to users in the form of SAS macros (Hannan and Murray 1996, Littell *et al.* 1996, Ch. 11). A useful evaluation of these different packages is provided by Zhou *et al.* (1999).

The major disadvantages of likelihood ratio tests are that they are computationally intensive and very tied to parametric assumptions. Of course, their optimal statistical properties in large samples somewhat compensate for these disadvantages. However, evidence from simulation studies (Shirley and Hickling 1981, Pack 1986, Donner *et al.* 1994) indicates that likelihood ratio tests may be unreliable in smaller samples (say, less than 40 clusters per group) and are not robust to departures from the assumed model.

**Generalized estimating equations approach**

The generalized estimating equations (GEE) approach, developed by Liang and Zeger (1986), can also be used to construct an extension of standard logistic regression which adjusts for the effect of clustering. In the absence of clustering, this approach reduces to that of standard logistic regression. A principal advantage of the GEE approach as compared with the parametric methods described above is that specification of an underlying distribution for the sample observations is not necessary.

Two distinct strategies are available to adjust for the effect of clustering using this approach. The first can be said to be model-based, as it requires the specification of a working correlation matrix which describes the pattern of correlation between responses of cluster members. For cluster randomization trials, the simplest assumption to make is that responses of cluster members are equally correlated, i.e. exchangeable. The resulting models will then be equivalent to those described by Williams (1982), at least when all covariates are measured at the cluster level. This is because the assumption of an exchangeable correlation matrix is then equivalent to assuming that the average correlation among cluster members does not vary among clusters.

As an example, consider a simple model to compare the prevalence of smokeless tobacco use in two intervention groups, based on the data provided in Table 6.2. This model would include only a single covariate indicating intervention group, as represented by a dummy variable. The validity of statistical inferences constructed using this strategy is assured provided the average intracluster correlation can be assumed to be constant across clusters, an assumption which also underlies the adjusted chi-square test procedure discussed at the beginning of this section.

The second strategy that may be used with GEE to adjust for the effect of clustering employs 'robust variance estimators' that are constructed using between-cluster information. These estimators consistently estimate the true variance even if the working correlation matrix is misspecified. Moreover, provided there are a large number of clusters, inferences obtained using robust variance estimators will become equivalent to those obtained using the model-based strategy when the working correlation matrix is correctly specified. An additional advantage is that relatively simple algebraic expressions are available to construct the resulting statistical inferences, at least when comparing responses of subjects from two or more independent groups (see Boos 1992).

Robust variance estimators have a relatively long history in survey research, well pre-dating the contributions of Liang and Zeger (1986). These earlier applications are based on the theory of ratio estimation (Lavange *et al.* 1994), as used in the test procedures proposed by Rao and Scott (1992). Implicit in this theory is the assumption of a fairly large number of clusters per intervention group (say, at least 20).

Significance tests based on the method of GEE can be obtained by comparing the square of the log odds ratio to its estimated variance. For the data in Table 6.2, the resulting model-based one degree of freedom chi-square test statistic is given by $\chi^2_{LZM} = 2.56$ ($p = 0.11$) (assuming an exchangeable working correlation matrix) with the robust version given by $\chi^2_{LZR} = 2.62$ ($p = 0.11$). Both versions were obtained using the procedure PROC GENMOD, available from the statistical package SAS (SAS Institute Inc. 1997). Test procedures based on GEE may also be conducted using the statistical package Stata (StataCorp 1997) or SUDAAN (Shah *et al.* 1996).

The relative capabilities of these different software packages are discussed by Ziegler and Gromping (1998). However, readers should be aware that robust variance estimators may be referred to in these packages as empirical or 'sandwich' estimators of variance.

In the absence of covariate adjustment, procedures simpler than GEE are likely to give similar results, and thus will often be preferred in practice. An important advantage of the GEE approach is that it can readily be extended to adjust for a combination of cluster-level and individual-level covariates, yielding consistent and asymptotically normally distributed estimators of regression coefficients. This feature was taken advantage of in the analysis of data arising from the church-based smoking cessation trial reported by Voorhees *et al.* (1996). These investigators randomized 22 churches to either an intensive culturally specific intervention or a minimal self-help intervention. Identified smokers were interviewed at baseline and at 1-year follow-up. Outcome variables included quit rates and 'positive progress along the stages of change', both of which were dichotomous. In comparing the intervention groups, the investigators chose to adjust for the influence of several variables, including age, gender and denomination. However, they recognized that since randomization was at the church level and the data were analysed at the individual level, standard multiple logistic regression analysis was not applicable. The correlation of responses within a church was therefore accounted for by applying the method of GEE (although the number of clusters per group is rather small to support the required assumptions). More detailed discussion of this approach as applied to data arising from cluster randomization trials can be found in Section 6.2.3.

#### 6.2.1.4 Summary of results

The results obtained from applying the procedures described above to the data in Table 6.2 are presented in Table 6.3. It is clear from this summary that the statistically significant result ($p = 0.03$) obtained from applying the standard Pearson chi-square statistic to the pooled data is highly misleading. The results from each of the other nine test statistics are clearly non-significant at the 5 per cent level. Thus there is no conclusive evidence from these data that the Smoke Free Generation intervention is effective in lowering the overall rate of tobacco use among these children, a conclusion also reached by Murray *et al.* (1992).

It should be noted that many of the difficulties in choosing among these test procedures essentially disappear when the cluster sizes are equal, i.e. $m_{ij} = m$, all $(i, j)$. In this case, we have $\chi^2_A = \chi^2_P/[1 + (m-1)\hat{\rho}]$. Moreover, it is straightforward to show that under these balanced conditions $\chi^2_A$ is closely approximated by $\chi^2_R$, $\chi^2_{LZM}$, $\chi^2_{LZR}$ and $t^2_u$, particularly under $H_0$. The differences among the various procedures become more pronounced as the variability among the cluster sizes increases.

**Table 6.3** Summary of test results obtained from a comparison of event rates in a completely randomized design

| Procedure | Test statistic | Two-sided $p$-value | Comment |
|---|---|---|---|
| Standard Pearson chi-square test for comparing proportions | $\chi^2_P = 4.69$ [a] | 0.03 | $p$-value biased downward in the presence of clustering. |
| Two-sample $t$-test | $t_u = -1.67$ (22 d.f.) | 0.11 | Required assumptions not strictly satisfied but very robust. |
| Wilcoxon rank sum test | $Z_{WT} = -1.41$<br>exact | 0.16<br>0.16 | Non-parametric test based on ranks |
| Two-sample permutation test | $Z_{PT} = -1.61$<br>exact | 0.11<br>0.11 | Non-parametric test based on observations |
| Direct adjustment of standard Pearson chi-square test | $\chi^2_A = 1.83$ | 0.18 | Reduces to standard Pearson chi-square test at $\hat{\rho} = 0$ |
| Ratio estimate chi-square test | $\chi^2_R = 2.08$ | 0.15 | Requires large numbers of clusters; well suited to non-randomized comparisons |
| Likelihood ratio test based on parametric modelling | $\chi^2_B = 1.81$<br>$\chi^2_{LN} = 1.97$ | 0.18<br>0.16 | Heavily model-dependent; computationally intensive |
| Generalized estimating equations | $\chi^2_{LZM} = 2.56$<br>$\chi^2_{LZR} = 2.62$ | 0.11<br>0.11 | Requires large numbers of clusters; can accommodate cluster-level and individual-level covariates; computationally intensive |

[a] All chi-square statistics presented in this table have one degree of freedom.

## 6.2.2 Confidence interval construction

It was mentioned in Chapter 1 that cluster randomization trials are frequently underpowered, and thus likely to be statistically non-significant even in the presence of substantial intervention effects. It is also well-known (e.g. Gardner and Altman 1986) that the interpretation of non-significant results from comparative trials is enhanced by their presentation in terms of confidence limits. An approximate two-sided $(1-\alpha)100$ per cent confidence interval about the effect of intervention estimated as a rate difference may be obtained as

$$(\hat{P}_1 - \hat{P}_2) \pm Z_{\alpha/2}\left[\frac{\hat{P}_1(1-\hat{P}_1)C_1}{M_1} + \frac{\hat{P}_2(1-\hat{P}_2)C_2}{M_2}\right]^{1/2}$$

where $Z_{\alpha/2}$ is the $(1-\alpha)100$ per cent two-sided critical value of the standard normal distribution. For the data in the present example, a 95 per cent confidence interval for $P_1 - P_2$ is given by

$$(0.043 - 0.062) \pm 1.96\left[\frac{(0.043)(0.957)2.536}{1341} + \frac{(0.062)(0.938)2.599}{1479}\right]^{1/2}$$
$$= (-0.045, 0.007)$$

At $\hat{\rho} = 0$ ($C_1 = C_2 = 1$), this expression reduces to the standard confidence interval about a rate difference (e.g. Armitage and Berry 1994, Section 4.8), but otherwise tends to be wider.

Note that the assumption of a common intracluster correlation $\rho$, although guaranteed under the null hypothesis of no intervention effect, may not be appropriate for confidence interval construction. In this case, separate estimates of $\rho$ may be used in computing the variance inflation factors $C_i$, $i = 1, 2$. However, these estimates would be reduced in precision as compared with the estimator $\hat{\rho}$, since the underlying sample sizes would be smaller.

The effect of intervention may alternatively be expressed in terms of the odds ratio $\Psi = P_1(1-P_2)/[P_2(1-P_1)]$. The sample odds ratio $\hat{\Psi} = \hat{P}_1(1-\hat{P}_2)/[\hat{P}_2(1-\hat{P}_1)]$ remains a consistent estimator of $\Psi$ in the presence of clustering, but, as with the rate difference, standard methods of confidence interval construction about $\hat{\Psi}$ must be modified. The estimated variance of $\ln(\hat{\Psi})$ is given (e.g. Donald and Donner 1987) by

$$\widehat{\text{Var}}(\ln\hat{\Psi}) = \frac{C_1}{M_1\hat{P}_1(1-\hat{P}_1)} + \frac{C_2}{M_2\hat{P}_2(1-\hat{P}_2)}$$

where 'ln' denotes logarithm to the base e. Hence approximate two-sided $(1-\alpha)$ 100 per cent confidence limits for $\Psi$ are given by

$$\left(e^{\ln\hat{\Psi} - Z_{\alpha/2}\sqrt{\widehat{\text{Var}}(\ln\hat{\Psi})}},\ e^{\ln\hat{\Psi} + Z_{\alpha/2}\sqrt{\widehat{\text{Var}}(\ln\hat{\Psi})}}\right)$$

At $\hat{\rho} = 0$, $\widehat{\text{Var}}(\ln\hat{\Psi})$ reduces to the variance estimate of a log odds ratio proposed by Woolf (1955).

For the data in the present example, the value of $\hat{\Psi}$ is given by

$$\frac{(0.043)(1-0.062)}{(0.062)(1-0.043)} = 0.68$$

and the 95 per cent confidence interval about $\hat{\Psi}$ by

$$(e^{\ln(0.68) - [1.96\sqrt{0.045\,96 + 0.030\,22}]}, e^{\ln(0.68) + [1.96\sqrt{0.045\,96 + 0.030\,22}]}) = (0.40, 1.17)$$

Odds ratio estimators and their associated confidence limits may also be obtained using any of the extensions of logistic regression described in the previous sections (e.g. beta-binomial, logistic-normal, GEE). For example, the GEE extension of logistic regression using a working exchangeable correlation matrix with a robust variance estimator provides an estimated odds ratio of 0.67 with a 95 per cent confidence interval given by (0.41, 1.09). Similar results can be obtained by using a model-based variance estimator or, alternatively, either a logistic-normal or beta-binomial extension of standard logistic regression. The closeness of the results obtained using these different approaches may be attributed in part to the small size of the pooled intracluster correlation coefficient (see Neuhaus 1992), as well as to the similarity of the intracluster correlation coefficients in the two intervention groups.

## 6.2.3 Adjusting for covariates

In Section 6.2.1, methods for comparing event rates were illustrated using data from the school-based smoking prevention trial reported by Murray *et al.* (1992). After adjusting for clustering, the impact of intervention on the use of smokeless tobacco was found to be not statistically significant. However, the methods presented in Section 6.2.1 did not account for the possibility that the observed results were due to chance imbalance on baseline covariates. Random assignment ensures that, on average, such covariates will be equally distributed or balanced across intervention groups. Nonetheless, in any one trial, some residual, but substantively important, imbalance may occur by chance. Such imbalance, of course, may also arise in trials randomizing individuals. However, for a given total number of individuals, the probability of an important imbalance will be higher in a trial randomizing clusters, owing to the smaller effective sample size. Provided the number of clusters is sufficiently large, multiple regression methods may be used to account for such imbalance, as well as to help increase the precision with which the intervention effect is estimated.

Baseline measures of student age and sex from this trial are provided in Table 6.4, separately by group for one of the experimental arms of the trial (Smoke Free Generation) and for the control arm (Existing Curriculum). These data indicate that both these covariates are balanced across the intervention groups. Cluster-level versions

**Table 6.4** Baseline measures for predictors of smokeless tobacco use

| | Smoke Free Generation | Existing Curriculum |
|---|---|---|
| Number of schools | 12 | 12 |
| Number of students | 1629 | 1747 |
| Mean age (years) | 11.8 | 11.8 |
| Sex (% male) | 50.6 | 52.5 |

of these variables (mean age per school, percentage of male students per school) are also well balanced.

As in our earlier analyses (see Table 6.2) we will restrict our attention here to the subgroup of 1341 experimental group children and 1479 control group children who provided information on smokeless tobacco use at follow-up. The internal validity of these analyses is not likely to be affected by attrition, since the rates of loss to follow-up are evenly distributed across intervention groups (Murray *et al.* 1992).

The impact of covariate adjustment on the estimated effect of intervention may be explored using the GEE extension of logistic regression. To describe the model underlying this procedure, some additional notation is required. Let $P_{ijl} = \Pr(Y_{ijl} = 1)$ denote the probability of using smokeless tobacco for the $l$th student, $l = 1, \ldots, m_{ij}$, from the $j$th cluster, $j = 1, \ldots, k_i$, of the $i$th intervention group, $i = 1, 2$. The odds ratio for the effect of intervention, adjusted for age and sex, can be obtained using the logistic regression model given by

$$\ln(P_{ijl}/[1 - P_{ijl}]) = \beta_0 + \beta_1 X_{ijl} + \beta_2 Age_{ijl} + \beta_3 Sex_{ijl} \tag{6.1}$$

where

$$X_{ijl} = \begin{cases} 1 & \text{if } i = 1 \text{ (experimental)} \\ 0 & \text{if } i = 2 \text{ (control)} \end{cases}$$

$$Sex_{ijl} = \begin{cases} 1 & \text{if male} \\ 0 & \text{if female} \end{cases}$$

and age (in years) is denoted by $Age_{ijl}$. The estimated odds ratio for the effect of intervention is then given by $\exp(\hat{\beta}_1)$. Inclusion of the variables $Age_{ijl}$ and $Sex_{ijl}$ in this model allows the effect of intervention to be adjusted for these baseline covariates. Estimated odds ratios for their independent effects are then obtained as $\exp(\hat{\beta}_2)$ and $\exp(\hat{\beta}_3)$ respectively.

This model can also be extended naturally to account for other quantitative or categorical covariates, analogous to the logistic regression analyses of data obtained from individually randomized trials (e.g. Rosner 1995, Section 11.14).

The results of fitting the model given by equation (6.1) using the SAS procedure PROC GENMOD are provided in Table 6.5, with statistical inferences constructed using a robust variance estimator with a working exchangeable correlation matrix. It is seen from these results that adjustment for age and sex results in a stronger observed effect of intervention, giving an adjusted odds ratio estimate of 0.65. As in our earlier analyses, however, the association is not statistically significant.

**Table 6.5** Estimated odds ratios, 95 per cent confidence intervals and two-sided *p*-value for smokeless tobacco use

| | Estimated odds ratio | 95% confidence interval | Two-sided *p*-value |
|---|---|---|---|
| Effect of intervention (SFG vs. EC) | 0.65 | (0.41, 1.04) | 0.07 |
| Age (years) | 1.24 | (0.60, 1.09) | 0.16 |
| Sex (male vs. female) | 31.86 | (14.51, 70.00) | <0.01 |

Covariate adjustment also resulted in a very modest reduction in the size of the estimated intracluster correlation coefficient, which remained close to 0.01. As noted in Section 5.2, reduction in the estimated intracluster correlation coefficient is most likely when adjustment is made for those covariates which most strongly account for between-cluster variation.

Investigators are often interested in conducting risk factor analyses which explore the association between selected baseline covariates and the study outcome variable. A complicating feature of such analyses in cluster randomization trials is that there may be different associations at the individual and cluster levels. For example, the results provided in Table 6.5 indicate that boys are much more likely to use smokeless tobacco than girls. However, a child's decision to use smokeless tobacco might not only be influenced by his or her sex but also by the overall proportion of boys in the school. This possibility can be explored using the strategy described by Neuhaus and Kalbfleisch (1998) in which the covariate $Sex_{ijl}$ is replaced by two new covariates. The within-cluster association between sex and smokeless tobacco use can be then assessed using the new covariate $(Sex_{ijl} - \overline{Sex}_{ij})$, where

$$\overline{Sex}_{ij} = \sum_{l=1}^{m_{ij}} Sex_{ijl}/m_{ij}$$

denotes the proportion of male students in each school. The possibility of a school-level (ecological) association may be assessed using the covariate $(\overline{Sex}_{ij} - \overline{Sex}_i)$, where

$$\overline{Sex}_i = \sum_{j-1}^{k_i} \sum_{l-1}^{m_{ij}} Sex_{ijl}/M_i$$

denotes the proportion of male students in the $i$th intervention group, $i = 1, 2$. Although the same strategy may be used for quantitative covariates as well (e.g. student age), the investigation of separate associations within and between clusters is only relevant for baseline covariates which vary within each cluster. Such investigations are therefore not required, and indeed are not possible, for covariates such as cluster size or intervention group.

Using data from the school-based trial reported by Murray *et al.* (1992), the observed associations of age and sex with smokeless tobacco use are qualitatively similar whether or not one allows for different associations at the individual and cluster levels. However, since there are only 12 clusters per intervention group, this conclusion should be interpreted cautiously, as would also be the case if mixed effects logistic regression models were used to analyse these data. The latter models have the advantage that they may more naturally be extended to account for associations at three or more levels (e.g. student, classroom, school).

Trials including large numbers of clusters can also be used to explore observed differences in the effect of intervention at the individual and cluster levels. For example, the effect of smokeless tobacco may be different for boys and girls within each school and, in addition, might have different effects depending on the proportion of boys in the school. We omit consideration of such interaction effects since, as noted, there are only 12 clusters per intervention group in this study.

### 6.2.4 Analysis strategies for trials with a small number of clusters per group

A special class of the studies considered here are community intervention trials, in which a fairly small number (often 10 or less) of relatively large units, such as medical practices, factories or entire cities, are allocated to different intervention groups. Koepsell *et al.* (1991, 1992) have discussed methodological issues arising in these studies, focusing on the case of a continuous response variable. When the response is dichotomous and the number of clusters is small, most of the methods discussed in Section 6.2.1, including the adjusted chi-square approach, the ratio estimator approach and the method of GEE, are no longer applicable, since the large sample approximations underlying these procedures become questionable. However, evidence suggests (e.g. Donner and Klar 1996, Hannan and Murray 1996) that the familiar two-sample *t*-test as applied to the cluster-specific event rates may be applied safely to data arising from community intervention trials with as few as three clusters per group, at least when there is little or no variation in cluster size. This is in contrast to the other approximate procedures discussed above, none of which will be trustworthy if the number of clusters per group is less than about 10. As discussed in Section 6.2.1.2, this remarkable robustness of the *t*-test to departures from the underlying assumptions of normality and homogeneity of variance has also been found by other investigators. However, the unattractive features of this procedure remain; in particular, the *t*-test does not yield results on a scale convenient for conducting further analyses.

An alternative approach to the *t*-test would be to obtain exact tests of significance using one of the non-parametric procedures discussed above, such as the Wilcoxon rank sum test or Fisher's permutation procedure. However, the limitation should be kept in mind that at least four clusters per group are required with these procedures to obtain a minimum two-sided *p*-value of 0.05.

These recommendations should not be taken as an endorsement of studies having a small number of clusters, since the limited power of these studies remains a problem. It follows that detailed attention to the problem of controlling type I error should not allow the investigator to lose sight of a possible type II error problem that distorts the proper interpretation of a non-significant result.

## 6.3 The matched-pair design

### 6.3.1 Comparison of proportions

The data from a matched-pair cluster randomization trial with a dichotomous outcome variable may be summarized in a series of $k$ $2 \times 2$ contingency tables of the form shown in Table 6.6.

The methods are discussed in the context of data arising from the London Hypertension Study (Bass *et al.* 1986, Donner 1987a), focusing for illustrative purposes on the subgroup of 5772 female patients aged 45 years or over. In particular, we investigate the effect of the experimental strategy on mortality from any cause in

**Table 6.6** Data arising from a matched-pair cluster randomization design

| | Experimental | Control | Total |
|---|---|---|---|
| Event | $a_{1j}$ | $a_{2j}$ | $r_{1j}$ |
| No event | $m_{1j} - a_{1j}$ | $m_{2j} - a_{2j}$ | $r_{2j}$ |
| Total | $m_{1j}$ | $m_{2j}$ | $m_j$ |

this patient subgroup. The relevant data for the 17 pairs of practices are shown in Table 6.7, in which the effect of the intervention may be summarized by the observed odds ratios $\hat{\Psi}_j = \hat{P}_{1j}(1 - \hat{P}_{2j})/[\hat{P}_{2j}(1 - \hat{P}_{1j})], j = 1, 2, \ldots, 17$, where $\hat{P}_{1j} = a_{1j}/m_{1j}$ and $\hat{P}_{2j} = a_{2j}/m_{2j}$ estimate the true proportions (event rates) $P_{1j}$ and $P_{2j}$ in the experimental and control groups, respectively. Our initial aim is to test the statistical significance of the intervention effect over all pairs of practices. More formally, we wish to test $H_0$: $\Psi = 1$, where $\Psi$ is the (assumed) common odds ratio. Since some of the test procedures below will be based on the observed differences $d_j = \hat{P}_{1j} - \hat{P}_{2j}, j = 1, 2, \ldots, 17$, we also present these quantities in Table 6.7.

**Table 6.7** Number of female patients aged 45 or over classified by intervention and outcome (Donner 1987a)

| | Experimental | Control | $\hat{P}_{1j}$ | $\hat{P}_{2j}$ | $\hat{\Psi}_j$ | $d_j$ |
|---|---|---|---|---|---|---|
| Death | 3 | 2 | 0.030 | 0.018 | 1.653 | 0.012 |
| No death | 98 | 108 | | | | |
| Death | 8 | 3 | 0.027 | 0.013 | 2.202 | 0.015 |
| No death | 287 | 237 | | | | |
| Death | 3 | 3 | 0.057 | 0.107 | 0.500 | −0.051 |
| No death | 50 | 25 | | | | |
| Death | 1 | 4 | 0.006 | 0.032 | 0.187 | −0.026 |
| No death | 163 | 122 | | | | |
| Death | 1 | 12 | 0.004 | 0.031 | 0.141 | −0.026 |
| No death | 223 | 376 | | | | |
| Death | 2 | 0 | 0.009 | 0.000 | – | 0.009 |
| No death | 211 | 80 | | | | |
| Death | 7 | 8 | 0.022 | 0.049 | 0.439 | −0.027 |
| No death | 311 | 156 | | | | |
| Death | 3 | 9 | 0.017 | 0.046 | 0.369 | −0.028 |
| No death | 169 | 187 | | | | |
| Death | 4 | 6 | 0.014 | 0.028 | 0.487 | −0.014 |
| No death | 285 | 208 | | | | |
| Death | 2 | 2 | 0.022 | 0.038 | 0.562 | −0.016 |
| No death | 89 | 50 | | | | |
| Death | 6 | 11 | 0.021 | 0.046 | 0.445 | −0.025 |
| No death | 277 | 226 | | | | |
| Death | 2 | 5 | 0.016 | 0.029 | 0.530 | −0.013 |
| No death | 126 | 167 | | | | |
| Death | 1 | 3 | 0.059 | 0.059 | 1.000 | 0.000 |
| No death | 16 | 48 | | | | |
| Death | 7 | 3 | 0.067 | 0.025 | 2.766 | 0.042 |
| No death | 97 | 115 | | | | |
| Death | 8 | 10 | 0.037 | 0.040 | 0.931 | −0.003 |
| No death | 207 | 241 | | | | |
| Death | 6 | 4 | 0.064 | 0.034 | 1.960 | 0.030 |
| No death | 88 | 115 | | | | |
| Death | 4 | 7 | 0.017 | 0.031 | 0.542 | −0.014 |
| No death | 233 | 221 | | | | |

#### *6.3.1.1 Standard Mantel–Haenszel chi-square test*

The Mantel–Haenszel one degree of freedom chi-square statistic for testing $H_0$: $\Psi = 1$ is given by

$$\chi^2_{\mathrm{MH}} = \frac{\left\{\sum_{j=1}^{k}(a_{1j} - m_{1j}r_{1j}/m_j)\right\}^2}{\sum_{j=1}^{k}\{m_{1j}m_{2j}r_{1j}(m_j - r_{1j})/[m_j^2(m_j - 1)]\}}$$

where $r_{1j} = a_{1j} + a_{2j}, j = 1, 2, \ldots, k$, and $m_j = m_{1j} + m_{2j}$, the total sample size for the $j$th table. Application of this statistic to the data in Table 6.7 is not valid, since the $a_{1j}$ and $a_{2j}$ cannot be regarded as having binomial distributions. This is because the lack of statistical independence among observations in the same cluster induces extra variability in the difference between $\hat{P}_{1j}$ and $\hat{P}_{2j}$, variability that is not accounted for in the test statistic. Thus the true level of significance associated with $\chi^2_{\mathrm{MH}}$ may be substantially greater than the nominal significance level if the clustering effect is ignored.

#### *6.3.1.2 Liang's test procedure*

Liang (1985) and Liang *et al.* (1986) have developed methodology for analysing $2 \times 2$ contingency tables when the binomial assumptions are relaxed. Although these authors emphasize its application to familial case–control studies, their methodology may also be applied to cluster randomization designs provided there are a substantial number of pairs (at least 25). Liang's one degree of freedom chi-square statistic is given by

$$\chi^2_{\mathrm{L}} = \frac{\left\{\sum_{j=1}^{k}(a_{1j} - m_{1j}r_{1j}/m_j)\right\}^2}{\sum_{j=1}^{k}(a_{1j} - m_{1j}r_{1j}/m_j)^2}$$

The numerator of $\chi^2_{\mathrm{L}}$ is identical to that of $\chi^2_{\mathrm{MH}}$, but the denominator reflects a variance term appropriate to the randomization of clusters within strata rather than individuals.

Applying Liang's statistic to the data in Table 6.7, we obtain $\chi^2_{\mathrm{L}} = 2.86$ ($p = 0.09$). This result provides some evidence of an intervention effect on mortality from any cause in this subgroup of patients, although it does not reach formal statistical significance at the 5 per cent level. Note, however, that the value of $\chi^2_{\mathrm{MH}}$ for these data is 4.85 ($p = 0.03$), illustrating how application of the Mantel–Haenszel test can lead to spurious statistical significance.

#### *6.3.1.3 Paired t-test*

A parametric approach is obtained by applying the standard paired $t$-test to the differences $d_j$, $j = 1, 2, \ldots, k$. Letting $\bar{d} = \sum_{j=1}^{k} d_j/k$ and $S_d^2 = \sum_{j=1}^{k}(d_j - \bar{d})^2/(k - 1)$, the paired $t$-statistic is given by $t_{\mathrm{p}} = (\bar{d}\sqrt{k})/S_d$, with $(k - 1)$ degrees of freedom. The main difficulty with this approach is that the underlying assumption of equal variances for the $d_j$ is clearly not satisfied for the present design, particularly if there is substantial variation in the cluster sizes. Application of the paired $t$-test also assumes that the $d_j$ can be regarded, at least approximately, as normally distributed. Empirical research (Korn 1984, Donner and Donald 1987, Gail *et al.* 1996) suggests, however, that $t_p$ is fairly robust to departures from these assumptions. For the data in Table 6.5, $t_p = -1.40$ ($p = 0.18$).

When cluster sizes are highly variable, some gain in power may be achieved using a weighted $t$-test, perhaps after transformation of the proportions $\hat{P}_{ij}$ to the arcsine or logit scale (Donner and Donald 1987). The latter transformation is particularly suitable for community-based trials involving large clusters, where simulation studies suggest that it may be safely applied to trials involving as few as six matched pairs (Donner and Donald 1987).

A paired $t$-test was used by Grosskurth *et al.* (1995) to test for the effect of intervention in their community trial examining the impact of improved treatment for sexually transmitted diseases (STDs) on HIV infection in rural Tanzania. This trial, first discussed in Chapter 1, involved six pairs of communities, matched on location and pre-existing STD rates. A random cohort of about 1000 adults aged 15–54 years from each community was surveyed at baseline and followed up 2 years later with respect to the incidence of HIV. Difference scores were calculated for each stratum as

$$d_j = \ln(\hat{P}_{1j}/\hat{P}_{2j}) = \ln(\hat{P}_{1j}) - \ln(\hat{P}_{2j})$$

Note that since the HIV incidence rates in this trial are relatively low (see Table 6.8), this transformation will give results similar to that based on a logit transform of the $\hat{P}_{ij}$.

The very high value of the matching correlation (0.94) achieved in the Tanzania trial attests to the success of the investigators in creating pairs of highly similar communities. Indeed, the statistically significant decrease in HIV incidence ($p < 0.01$) which may be attributed to the effect of intervention would not have been achieved had the matching been ignored in the analysis.

Investigators may find it counter-intuitive (and perhaps depressing) that a trial enrolling thousands of subjects leads to a primary analysis consisting essentially of a paired $t$-test with limited degrees of freedom. However, this is inevitable when between-stratum information is used to estimate error variability, as must be the case for this design. Increasing the amount of within-stratum information by increasing the sizes of the matched clusters will not increase the degrees of freedom available

**Table 6.8** HIV incidence rates in experimental and control communities (Grosskurth *et al.* 1995)

| Community pair | Experimental | Control |
|---|---|---|
| 1. Rural | 5/568 (0.9%) | 10/702 (1.4%) |
| 2. Islands | 4/766 (0.5%) | 7/833 (0.8%) |
| 3. Roadside | 17/650 (2.6%) | 20/630 (3.2%) |
| 4. Lakeshore | 13/734 (1.8%) | 23/760 (3.0%) |
| 5. Lakeshore | 4/732 (0.5%) | 12/782 (1.5%) |
| 6. Rural | 5/699 (1.2%) | 10/693 (1.4%) |
| Overall | 48/4149 (1.2%) | 82/4400 (1.9%) |

for testing the effect of intervention. It will, of course, increase the power of the test by adding to the precision with which the effect of intervention is estimated within strata. Nonetheless, this impact will be small if the between-stratum variability remains relatively large in magnitude.

#### 6.3.1.4 Non-parametric approaches

Classical non-parametric approaches could also be used for testing $H_0$. These have the advantage of avoiding distributional assumptions, such as normality, but as a consequence suffer from reduced power. They also do not take into account the variable cluster sizes that characterize most trials. One such approach is the Wilcoxon signed rank test as applied to the $d_j = \hat{P}_{1j} - \hat{P}_{2j}$, based on the ranks of the $d_j$ rather than on their actual values. Although the null distribution of the appropriate test statistic has been tabulated in exact form, a normal approximation will be adequate provided that the number of pairs is at least 15 (counting only the non-zero $d_j$ values). The test is performed by first ranking the absolute values of the $d_j$, with the smallest rank assigned the rank 1. Strata having identical absolute values of $d_j$ are assigned the mean rank as described by Rosner (1995, Section 12.3). Letting $T$ denote the sum of ranks for those strata having $d_j > 0$, the test procedure is performed by comparing the value of $T$ with the corresponding sum of ranks expected under $H_0$. An approximate normal deviate test statistic is then given by

$$Z_{WS} = \frac{T - \dfrac{k(k+1)}{4}}{\sqrt{\dfrac{k(k+1)(2k+1)}{24}}}$$

where $k$ now denotes the number of strata with non-zero values of $d_j$. Applying this procedure to the $k = 16$ non-zero values of $d_j$ shown in Table 6.7, we obtain $T = 41$ and $Z_{WS} = -1.40$ ($p = 0.16$). An exact $p$-value for testing $H_0$ can be computed using Proc-StatXact (Mehta and Patel 1997), and is given for these data by 0.17. Provided there are no tied values (as is the case here), exact $p$-values may also be obtained using standard tables (e.g. Rosner 1995, Appendix Table 12).

A version of this procedure was used in the hypertension screening and management trial described in Section 1.1 (Bass *et al.* 1986), where it was regarded as necessary first to adjust for observed differences between the two intervention groups with respect to age and smoking status. This was done by computing adjusted event rates for each individual practice using the well-known method of direct standardization (Armitage and Berry 1994, Section 12.6). The resulting differences in adjusted rates between the experimental and control groups was computed for each matched pair and the Wilcoxon signed rank test applied to these differences.

An alternative to this procedure is Fisher's one-sample permutation test, which uses the magnitude of the $d_j$ as well as their ranks. Under the null hypothesis that the intervention has no effect, the event rates within each matched pair would remain the same even if the labels 'experimental' and 'control' were interchanged. Since the assignment of these labels may be regarded as random under $H_0$, there are a total of $2^k$ equally likely permutations that can arise under these rearrangements. The value of $\bar{d} = \sum_{j=1}^{k} d_j/k$ actually observed can then be compared with its probability distribution as tabulated over all such outcomes. A value which is too 'extreme' would lead to rejection of $H_0$. This generally requires some fairly heavy computation. However, since the $d_j$ are approximately distributed under $H_0$ with mean zero and variance $\sum_{j=1}^{k}(d_j^2/k)$, a simple form of this test is often used in practice, where

$$Z_{PS} = \sum_{j=1}^{k} d_j \Big/ \sqrt{\sum_{j=1}^{k} d_j^2}$$

is referred to tables of the standard normal distribution. For the data in Table 6.7, $Z_{PS} = -1.36$ ($p = 0.17$). An exact $p$-value for the one sample permutation test may be obtained using the statistical package Proc-StatXact (Mehta and Patel 1997), given for these data by 0.19. Note that this result is virtually identical to that obtained using the paired $t$-test even though application of the permutation test requires no model-based assumptions. One limitation of the exact permutation test is that a minimum of six pairs of clusters is required to obtain a two-sided $p$-value of less than 0.05.

Gail *et al.* (1992) provide a detailed discussion of permutation tests as applied to the design and analysis of the COMMIT community intervention trial. A further example of this procedure is given by Maritz and Jarrett (1983), who applied the statistic $Z_{PS}$ to an observational comparison of cancer mortality rates within 32 pairs of cities, where one city had a 'high' level of fluoride content in the drinking water, and the other had a 'low' level.

### 6.3.1.5 Summary of results

There are some interesting relationships between the various test statistics described above. For example, it may be shown that $t_P = Z_{PS}(k-1)^{1/2}/(k - Z_{PS}^2)^{1/2}$, and that whenever $t_P$ has a large sample distribution, the one-sample permutation statistic $Z_{PS}$ has the same distribution (Cressie 1980). This result affirms the validity of the paired $t$-test in large samples even though the underlying differences $d_j$ are not identically distributed normal variates. It also shows that the power of the permutation test approaches that of the paired $t$-test as the number of pairs increases. The permutation test is also closely related to Liang's statistic $\chi_L^2$ and to the Wilcoxon signed rank test. Thus (i) $\chi_L^2$ can be regarded as a weighted version of the permutation test (Donner 1987b), and (ii) the signed rank test is simply the permutation test applied to the ranks of the $d_j$.

The results of the various test procedures presented in this section are summarized in Table 6.9. This summary reflects the similarity in results to be expected from the various methods when the number of strata is reasonably large (say $k \geqslant 15$). The only statistically significant result was obtained using the (invalid) Mantel–Haenszel chi-square statistic. The results from the other six procedures are clearly non-significant at the 5 per cent level. Thus there is no conclusive evidence that the hypertension screening programme was effective at reducing female mortality. A final point to remember is that approximate statistical inferences constructed using either Liang's statistic or the Wilcoxon signed rank test should be avoided when there is a small number of strata. It may be preferable in this case to rely on exact statistical inferences that are constructed using permutation tests, or, alternatively, to perform a paired $t$-test after transformation of the event rates to the logistic

**Table 6.9** Summary of test results obtained from a comparison of event rates in a matched-pair design (Donner 1987a)

| Procedure | Test statistic | Two-sided $p$-value | Comment |
|---|---|---|---|
| Mantel–Haenszel chi-square | $\chi^2_{MH} = 4.85$ (1 d.f.) | 0.03 | $p$-value biased downward in the presence of clustering |
| Wilcoxon signed rank test | $Z_{WS} = -1.40$ | 0.16 | Non-parametric test based on ranks |
| | exact | 0.17 | |
| One-sample permutation test | $Z_{PS} = -1.36$ | 0.17 | Non-parametric test based on observations |
| | exact | 0.19 | |
| Liang chi-square | $\chi^2_L = 2.86$ (1 d.f.) | 0.09 | Weighted version of $Z_{PS}$ that takes into account cluster sizes |
| Paired $t$-test | $t_P = -1.40$ (16 d.f.) | 0.18 | Required assumptions not strictly satisfied but very robust |

scale (Donner and Donald 1987). However, as noted in Section 6.2.4, proper attention to considerations of statistical power at the design stage should help to avoid the likelihood that trials of very small size will be mounted.

## 6.3.2 Confidence interval construction

Although the Mantel–Haenszel chi-square statistic $\chi^2_{MH}$ is not valid for matched-pair cluster randomization designs, the associated Mantel–Haenszel estimator $\hat{\Psi}_{MH}$ of an assumed common odds ratio $\Psi$ remains consistent, i.e. $\hat{\Psi}_{MH}$ will approach the value of this parameter in large samples. Using the present notation, $\hat{\Psi}_{MH}$ may be computed for the data in Table 6.7 as

$$\hat{\Psi}_{MH} = \frac{\sum_{j=1}^{k} a_{1j}(m_{2j} - a_{2j})/m_j}{\sum_{j=1}^{k} a_{2j}(m_{1j} - a_{1j})/m_j} = \frac{\sum_{j=1}^{k} U_j}{\sum_{j=1}^{k} V_j} = 0.70$$

Provided the number of pairs (strata) is fairly large, the large sample variance of $\hat{\Psi}_{MH}$ may be estimated from between-stratum information, and is given in this case (Liang 1985) by

$$\widehat{\text{Var}}(\hat{\Psi}_{MH}) = \sum_{j=1}^{k} (U_j - \hat{\Psi}_{MH} V_j)^2 \Big/ \left[\sum_{j=1}^{k} V_j\right]^2$$

However, the sampling distribution of $\hat{\Psi}_{MH}$ tends to be severely non-normal, and thus confidence interval construction about this estimator is usually based on the distribution of its logarithm. The variance of $\ln(\hat{\Psi}_{MH})$ may be estimated by $\widehat{\text{Var}}(\ln \hat{\Psi}_{MH}) = \widehat{\text{Var}}(\hat{\Psi}_{MH})/(\hat{\Psi}_{MH})^2$. Thus approximate two-sided $(1 - \alpha)100$ per cent confidence limits about $\Psi$ are given, after approximate transformation, by

$$\exp\{\ln(\hat{\Psi}_{MH}) \pm Z_{\alpha/2}[\widehat{\text{Var}}(\ln \hat{\Psi}_{MH})^{1/2}]\}$$

Application of these limits in practice requires a large number of strata (say $\geqslant 15$). For the data in Table 6.7, approximate 95 per cent confidence limits for $\Psi$ are given by

$$\exp[\ln(0.70) \pm 1.96(0.0352)^{1/2}] = (0.48, 1.01)$$

Greater efficiency may be obtained using weighted versions of the Mantel–Haenszel odds ratio estimator as shown by Donner and Hauck (1988, 1989). Inference procedures may alternatively be conducted using an extension of Woolf's odds ratio estimator (Woolf 1955, Fleiss 1981, Section 10.2, Donner and Klar 1993). These procedures, based on a weighted average of the logarithms of the stratum-specific odds ratios, are particularly suitable for community-based trials involving a relatively small number of large strata. In this sense, they complement inference procedures based on the Mantel–Haenszel estimator.

## 6.3.3 Adjusting for covariates

The prematching of experimental units on prognostic factors potentially related to outcome is a commonly used strategy for ensuring balance on these factors. However, substantial imbalances between groups on other important factors can still arise, as is the case in all randomized studies. In this section, we discuss methods of adjusting for such cluster-level covariates.

A simple method of dealing with a small number of categorical covariates would be to stratify on these factors within each of the original $k$ pairs (strata). Separate summary tables could then be constructed for each combination of confounders and the methods above directly applied. This approach, however, becomes very unwieldy as the number of covariates increases.

A more efficient approach to controlling for several cluster-level covariates in matched-pair designs is to adopt the log-linear model given by

$$\ln(\Psi_j) = \alpha + \beta_1 Z_{1j} + \beta_2 Z_{2j} + \ldots + \beta_h Z_{hj} \tag{6.2}$$

where $\Psi_j$ is the odds ratio associated with stratum $j$, $j = 1, 2, \ldots, k$, and the $Z_{uj}$, $u = 1, 2, \ldots, h$, are appropriately selected covariates.

Breslow (1976) investigated this model for the case in which $a_{1j}$ and $a_{2j}$ are binomial variates, $j = 1, 2, \ldots, k$, as would be the case if individuals rather than clusters were randomized within each strata. Liang *et al.* (1986), however, have generalized Breslow's methodology to deal with sampling models in which the binomial assumption is relaxed, and which can be applied to the design considered here. We now apply this methodology to data arising from the London Hypertension Study (Bass *et al.* 1986).

Information on potential confounding factors in this study was obtained from a one-page questionnaire that recorded alcohol consumption, smoking habits, weight and height. We may first be interested in knowing whether these risk factors are equally distributed in the experimental and control groups among female patients aged 45 or over. Table 6.10 shows that the percentage of current smokers is somewhat higher among experimental patients than among control patients, while the

**Table 6.10** Percentage of female patients aged 45 or over reporting various risk factors (Donner 1987a)

| | Experimental group | Control group |
|---|---|---|
| % Current smoker | 28.8 | 23.3 |
| % Non-drinker | 25.3 | 28.8 |
| % Obese[a] | 41.3 | 46.1 |

[a] Body mass index: weight/height$^2$ > 25 kg/m$^2$.

percentage of non-drinkers and obese patients is somewhat lower. It is therefore of interest to know whether the intervention effect is statistically significant after adjusting for these differences. This is most easily accomplished by defining the covariates $Z_{uj}$, $u = 1, 2, 3$ as the difference in covariate $u$ between practices in the $j$th stratum. For example, $Z_{1j}$ is calculated as the difference between the percentage of current smokers in the experimental and control group practices belonging to stratum $j$. Thus if the two practices in the $j$th stratum are identical on all covariates, i.e. $Z_{uj} = 0$, $u = 1, 2, \ldots, h$, the model in equation (6.2) reduces to $\ln(\Psi_j) = \alpha$. This implies that $\exp(\alpha)$ may be regarded as the odds ratio after adjusting for the covariates, and that testing $H_0$: $\alpha = 0$ is equivalent to testing whether this odds ratio is equal to 1. In the context of the present example, testing $H_0$: $\alpha = 0$ is equivalent to testing whether the odds ratio associated with the experimental intervention is equal to unity after allowing for group differences with respect to smoking, drinking and obesity.

For the example here, the estimate of $\alpha$ is obtained as $\hat{\alpha} = -0.393$, with estimated standard error given by $\widehat{\text{SE}}(\hat{\alpha}) = 0.208$. Thus, a large sample test of $H_0$: $\alpha = 0$ is obtained by referring the ratio $-0.393/0.208 = -1.89$ to tables of the standard normal distribution. The $p$-value for this test is 0.06, while the estimate of the adjusted odds ratio is given by $\exp(-0.393) = 0.68$; 95 per cent confidence limits for the adjusted odds ratio may be computed as $\exp[-0.393 \pm 1.96(0.208)]$ or $(0.45, 1.01)$. It is worth noting that if $\beta_1 = \beta_2 \ldots = \beta_h = 0$ in equation (6.2), the estimator of the common odds ratio $\exp(\alpha)$ given by this estimation technique will be the Mantel–Haenszel estimator. For this reason, this procedure can be regarded as an extension of the Mantel–Haenszel test that controls for cluster-level baseline covariates. This technique must be used cautiously, not only because there is no unique way to model individual-level covariates at the cluster level, but also because cluster-level adjustment does not necessarily imply adjustment at the individual level (Morgenstern 1998), an example of the ecological fallacy.

## 6.4 The stratified design

As discussed in Section 3.6, the stratified design allows the replication of clusters in at least some combinations of intervention and stratum, and hence a valid estimate of $\rho$ can be directly calculated. This in turn permits the standard Mantel–Haenszel test statistic to be adjusted for clustering in a straightforward manner.

Suppose that the data layout at the analysis stage is given by Table 6.11, where the number of subjects contributed by the experimental group and control group clusters in stratum $j$ are denoted by $M_{1j}$, $M_{2j}$, respectively, with $M_j = M_{1j} + M_{2j}$. The

**Table 6.11** Data layout for a stratified cluster randomization design

| Stratum | Intervention | Number of clusters | Number of subjects classified as success | Number of subjects |
|---|---|---|---|---|
| 1 | Experimental | $n_{11}$ | $A_{11}$ | $M_{11}$ |
| | Control | $n_{21}$ | $A_{21}$ | $M_{21}$ |
| | Total | | $A_1$ | $M_1$ |
| 2 | Experimental | $n_{12}$ | $A_{12}$ | $M_{12}$ |
| | Control | $n_{22}$ | $A_{22}$ | $M_{22}$ |
| | Total | | $A_2$ | $M_2$ |
| ⋮ | | | ⋮ | ⋮ |
| $S$ | Experimental | $n_{1S}$ | $A_{1S}$ | $M_{1S}$ |
| | Control | $n_{2S}$ | $A_{2S}$ | $M_{2S}$ |
| | Total | | $A_S$ | $M_S$ |

corresponding number of subjects classified as a 'success' are denoted by $A_{1j}$, $A_{2j}$, with $A_j = A_{1j} + A_{2j}$. Let $n_{1jm}$, $n_{2jm}$ denote the number of experimental and control group clusters in stratum $j$ having exactly $m$ subjects. The required adjustment to the standard Mantel–Haenszel procedure depends on clustering correction factors defined for the experimental and control groups, respectively, as

$$C_{1j} = \left[\sum_m m[1 + (m-1)\hat{\rho}]n_{1jm}\right] / M_{1j}$$

and

$$C_{2j} = \left[\sum_m m[1 + (m-1)\hat{\rho}]n_{2jm}\right] / M_{2j}$$

where $\hat{\rho}$ is the estimated intracluster correlation coefficient, and the summation is taken over all clusters of size $m$. One simple method for obtaining this estimate is to first compute the standard estimator of intracluster correlation in each stratum, as described in Section 6.2.1. The overall estimator $\hat{\rho}$ may then be obtained as the average of these separate estimators. An alternative estimator, likely to be more efficient if the data are highly imbalanced, could be developed using nested analysis of variance (Dunn and Clark 1987, Ch. 6).

The required generalization of the Mantel–Haenszel procedure is given (e.g. Donner 1998) by

$$\chi^2_{\text{MHA}} = \frac{\left[\sum_{j=1}^{S} \frac{A_{1j}(M_{2j} - A_{2j}) - A_{2j}(M_{1j} - A_{1j})}{M_{1j}C_{2j} + M_{2j}C_{1j}}\right]^2}{\sum_{j=1}^{S} \frac{M_{1j}M_{2j}A_j(M_j - A_j)}{(M_{1j}C_{2j} + M_{2j}C_{1j} - 1)M_j^2}}$$

Let $\Psi$ denote the intervention odds ratio, assumed constant across strata. Under $H_0$: $\Psi = 1$, $\chi^2_{\text{MHA}}$ has an approximate chi-square distribution with one degree of freedom.

It is easy to verify that the adjusted statistic $\chi^2_{\text{MHA}}$ is identical to the standard Mantel–Haenszel test statistic if $C_{1j} = C_{2j} = 1$, $j = 1, 2, \ldots, S$. If all clusters are of the same size $m$, then we also have $\chi^2_{\text{MHA}} \simeq \chi^2_{\text{MH}}/[1 + (m-1)\hat{\rho}]$, showing that $\chi^2_{\text{MH}}$

is spuriously inflated by a factor of size $[1 + (m - 1)\hat{\rho}]$ if within-cluster dependencies are ignored.

The confidence interval methods presented in Section 6.3 for the matched-pair design may also be applied to the stratified design. In particular, if the number of strata is reasonably large (say $\geqslant 20$), methods based on the Mantel–Haenszel estimator $\hat{\Psi}_{MH}$ may be used (Donner and Klar 1993). If the number of strata is small, but there are a large number of observations in each stratum, it would be preferable to use methods based on logarithms of the stratum-specific odds ratios (e.g. see Donner 1998).

Statistical analyses for the stratified design may also be conducted using GEE or other extensions of logistic regression. Unlike the adjusted Mantel–Haenszel procedure, the use of GEE in this context allows adjustment for individual-level as well as cluster-level covariates, with the variation in event rates among strata accommodated using indicator variables. Thus trials with $S$ strata would include $S - 1$ indicator variables, as commonly done in the construction of standard logistic regression models.

For trials with a relatively small number of clusters per intervention group, it may be prudent to restrict analyses to the cluster level. An added advantage of this restriction would be that exact statistical inferences could be constructed using stratified permutation tests, where all possible reallocations of clusters are considered separately by stratum. These analyses can be conducted using readily available computer programs such as Proc-StatXact (Mehta and Patel 1997). Other extensions of standard non-parametric rank tests for stratified samples are discussed by Lehmann (1975, pp. 132–141) and Fry and Lee (1988).

# 7

# Analysis of quantitative outcomes

The purpose of this chapter is to describe methods of analysis applicable to cluster randomization trials where the study outcome is quantitative. The methods we describe may therefore be used to analyse data from trials which include study outcomes such as weight, body temperature or summary scores from standardized questionnaires. Only limited attention is given to the scale (e.g. ratio, interval, ordinal) on which a quantitative outcome is measured, leaving investigators to decide whether estimates of treatment effects are interpretable for the specified outcome. We note, however, that tests of hypotheses constructed using parametric procedures are often valid for ordinal outcomes as well (e.g. Heeren and D'Agostino 1987). Additional discussion of ordinal outcome data is provided in Chapter 8. Readers interested in a more general discussion of measurement scales may wish to consult Hand (1996).

The discussion in this chapter is presented separately by study design. Methods for the completely randomized design are described in Section 7.1, while methods for the matched-pair and stratified designs are presented in Sections 7.2 and 7.3, respectively.

## 7.1 The completely randomized design

### 7.1.1 Comparison of two means

The primary aim of many trials is to compare two groups of subjects with respect to their mean values on a quantitative outcome variable $Y$, assumed to have an approximate normal distribution. This goal may be formalized by establishing the null hypothesis $H_0: \mu_1 = \mu_2$, where $\mu_1$ and $\mu_2$ are the underlying means of $Y$ in the experimental and control groups, respectively. All the procedures discussed may be extended in a natural way to the comparison of more than two groups.

Suppose that $k_i$ clusters have been allocated to group $i$ ($i = 1, 2$), with $Y_{ijl}$ denoting the response of subject $l$ in the $j$th cluster of group $i$. Furthermore, let $\overline{Y}_{ij}$ denote the mean response computed over all $m_{ij}$ subjects in this cluster. Then the mean of $Y_{ijl}$ as computed over all subjects in group $i$ may be written as

$$\overline{Y}_i = \frac{\sum_{j=1}^{k_i} m_{ij}\overline{Y}_{ij}}{\sum_{j=1}^{k_i} m_{ij}}$$

where $\overline{Y}_1 - \overline{Y}_2$ estimates the population mean difference $\mu_1 - \mu_2$. We further denote the total number of individuals in the study by

$$M = \sum_{i=1}^{2}\sum_{j=1}^{k_i} m_{ij}$$

the total number of clusters by

$$K = \sum_{i=1}^{2} k_i$$

and the mean cluster size by $\overline{m} = M/K$.

Testing the difference $\overline{Y}_1 - \overline{Y}_2$ for statistical significance requires the computation of a standard error that takes into account the randomization by cluster. This is done by first quantifying the degree of dependence within clusters, as measured by the intracluster correlation coefficient.

Letting

$$\overline{m}_{Ai} = \sum_{j=1}^{k_i} \frac{m_{ij}^2}{M_i}$$

where

$$M_i = \sum_{j=1}^{k_i} m_{ij}$$

is the total number of individuals in group $i$, the 'analysis of variance' estimator of the intracluster correlation coefficient $\rho$ is defined (Dunn and Clark 1987, pp. 116–119) as

$$\hat{\rho} = \frac{\text{MSC} - \text{MSW}}{\text{MSC} + (m_0 - 1)\text{MSW}}$$

where

$$\text{MSC} = \sum_{i=1}^{2}\sum_{j=1}^{k_i} m_{ij}\frac{(\overline{Y}_{ij} - \overline{Y}_i)^2}{K-2}$$

$$\text{MSW} = \sum_{i=1}^{2}\sum_{j=1}^{k_i}\sum_{l=1}^{m_{ij}} \frac{(Y_{ijl} - \overline{Y}_{ij})^2}{M-K}$$

and

$$m_0 = \frac{M - \sum_{i=1}^{2} \overline{m}_{Ai}}{K - 2}$$

This estimator may be written equivalently as $\hat{\rho} = S_A^2/(S_A^2 + S_W^2)$, where $S_A^2 = (\text{MSC} - \text{MSW})/m_0$ and $S_W^2 = \text{MSW}$ denote sample estimates of $\sigma_A^2$ and $\sigma_W^2$, the between- and within-cluster components of variance, respectively. Note also that the estimator $\hat{\rho}$ pools observations across clusters in both groups, and thus assumes a common value of the population intracluster correlation $\rho$. However, if clusters are randomly allocated to the two groups, then this assumption is guaranteed under $H_0$, as previously discussed in Chapter 6. Also note that in the case of a single sample, i.e. when $\hat{\rho}$ is computed over the clusters in one group only, this estimator reduces to the standard estimator of an intracluster correlation coefficient obtained from a one-way analysis of variance, as given by equation (1.2).

The mean square errors MSC and MSW measure the variation in response among and within clusters, respectively. If responses on subjects within a cluster are no more similar than responses on subjects within different clusters, then MSC = MSW and $\hat{\rho} = 0$. If all responses within a cluster are identical, then MSW = 0 and $\hat{\rho} = 1$.

The methods of analysis will be illustrated using data from a worksite intervention trial designed, in part, to evaluate a weight loss health promotion programme (source not cited due to reasons of confidentiality). Of the 32 participating worksites, 16 were randomly assigned to receive onsite weight loss instruction while the remaining worksites were assigned to a control group. For purposes of illustration, analyses are limited here to a comparison of cross-sectional samples of 4134 employees for whom body mass index (a measure of obesity) was available two years following the intervention. The mean body mass index at 2 years is given by $\overline{Y}_1 = 25.62\,\text{kg/m}^2$ for the $M_1 = 1929$ subjects in the experimental group, and by $\overline{Y}_2 = 25.98\,\text{kg/m}^2$ for the $M_2 = 2205$ subjects in the control group.

#### 7.1.1.1 Standard two sample t-test

We begin our comparison of methods by considering the standard two-sample $t$-test, which is not applicable to this design unless adjusted for the effects of clustering. Application of this statistic to testing $H_0\colon \mu_1 = \mu_2$ yields

$$t = \frac{\overline{Y}_1 - \overline{Y}_2}{\sqrt{\dfrac{(M_1 - 1)S_1^2 + (M_2 - 1)S_2^2}{M - 2}\left(\dfrac{1}{M_1} + \dfrac{1}{M_2}\right)}}$$

$$= \frac{25.62 - 25.98}{\sqrt{\dfrac{(1929 - 1)22.4 + (2205 - 1)24.6}{4134 - 2}\left(\dfrac{1}{1929} + \dfrac{1}{2205}\right)}}$$

$$= -2.37 \quad (p = 0.02)$$

where

$$S_i^2 = \sum_{j=1}^{k_i} \sum_{l=1}^{m_{ij}} \frac{(Y_{ijl} - \overline{Y}_i)^2}{M_i - 1}$$

The resulting $p$-value is almost certainly too small, as it ignores the effects of clustering. The standard assumption that $t$ has $(M_1 - 1) + (M_2 - 1) = 1928 + 2204 = 4132$ degrees of freedom is also violated here.

The magnitude of the bias associated with $t$ increases with both the value of $\rho$ and the average cluster size. For clusters of fixed size $m$, and ignoring issues of degrees of freedom, the bias is given by the square root of the variance inflation factor, i.e. by $\sqrt{1 + (m - 1)\rho}$.

### 7.1.1.2 Cluster-level analyses

Cluster-level analyses were introduced in Section 6.2.1.2 for binary outcome data as obtained from trials using completely randomized designs. These methods may be directly applied to the unweighted mean responses by replacing $\hat{P}_{ij}$ with $\overline{Y}_{ij}$, $i = 1, 2,\ j = 1, 2, \ldots, k_i$. For example, a two-sample $t$-test could be used to test $H_0\colon \mu_1 = \mu_2$ using the 32 worksite means from the trial referred to previously. This yields an approximate two-sided $p$-value of 0.24 with 30 degrees of freedom. In general, this statistic will provide exact $p$-values only when the cluster sizes are equal.

The parametric assumptions underlying the $t$-test may be avoided by adopting a non-parametric procedure. A particularly useful class of non-parametric procedures are permutation or randomization tests, which use the actual values of the observations rather than only their ranks. As discussed in Chapter 6, these tests tend to be more powerful than rank tests, although they are less powerful than parametric procedures such as the $t$-test when the assumptions underlying the latter are satisfied.

Returning to the worksite intervention trial, an exact two-sided $p$-value of 0.42 is obtained using the Wilcoxon rank sum test, while applying the two-sample permutation test to the cluster-specific mean responses yields an exact two-sided $p$-value of 0.24. Both $p$-values were calculated using Proc-StatXact (Mehta and Patel 1997).

### 7.1.1.3 Individual-level analyses

In this section we consider two alternative methods for conducting individual-level analyses of quantitative outcome data. The first approach is based on a simple extension of the standard two-sample $t$-test. A more flexible but computationally intensive mixed effects linear repression approach is also described.

#### Adjusted two-sample *t*-test

An attractive feature of the estimator $\hat{\rho}$ is that it may be directly applied to obtaining an appropriate standard error for testing $H_0\colon \mu_1 = \mu_2$. Denote the overall pooled variance by $S_p^2 = S_A^2 + S_W^2$, where $S_p^2$ estimates the parameter $\sigma^2 = \sigma_A^2 + \sigma_W^2$, assumed to be constant across all subject scores.

The estimated standard error of $\overline{Y}_1 - \overline{Y}_2$ is then given by

$$\widehat{\mathrm{SE}}(\overline{Y}_1 - \overline{Y}_2) = S_P \left[ \frac{C_1}{M_1} + \frac{C_2}{M_2} \right]^{1/2}$$

where

$$C_i = \sum_{j=1}^{k_i} m_{ij} \frac{1 + (m_{ij} - 1)\hat{\rho}}{M_i} = 1 + (\overline{m}_{Ai} - 1)\hat{\rho}$$

is the variance inflation factor computed for group $i$ ($i = 1, 2$) (Donner and Klar 1993).

A test of $H_0{:}\,\mu_1 = \mu_2$ is now obtained by referring the approximate statistic $t_A = (\overline{Y}_1 - \overline{Y}_2)/\widehat{SE}(\overline{Y}_1 - \overline{Y}_2)$ to tables of the $t$-distribution with $K - 2$ degrees of freedom. At $\hat{\rho} = 0$, this test procedure reduces to the standard $t$-test for comparing two independent means.

An approximate two-sided $(1 - \alpha)100$ per cent confidence interval for the population mean difference $\mu_1 - \mu_2$ is given by

$$(\overline{Y}_1 - \overline{Y}_2) \pm t_{\alpha/2}\widehat{SE}(\overline{Y}_1 - \overline{Y}_2)$$

where $t_{\alpha/2}$ is the $(1 - \alpha)100$ per cent two-sided critical value of the $t$-distribution with $K - 2$ degrees of freedom.

The assumption of a common intracluster correlation may not hold when constructing confidence limits for the population mean difference. Although procedures based on large sample theory are available to construct tests for a common intracluster correlation (e.g. Mian and Shoukri 1997), most cluster randomization trials will not have sufficient power to adequately test such hypotheses. Thus a statistically non-significant result from such a test cannot, in general, be taken to imply that there is no difference in the degree of intracluster correlation across groups. As an alternative, investigators might prefer to conduct a sensitivity analysis that examines the effect of relaxing the assumptions of a common variance and intracluster correlation when constructing a confidence interval for $\mu_1 - \mu_2$. The reliability of the trial conclusions will be enhanced to the extent that they remain stable across different sets of assumptions.

We illustrate these methods using data from the worksite intervention trial. The estimated variance components were obtained as $S_A^2 = 0.50$ and $S_W^2 = 23.0$ using the ANOVA option of the SAS procedure PROC VARCOMP. Similarly the estimated pooled variance $S_P^2 = 0.50 + 23.0$, the estimated intracluster correlation coefficient is given by $\hat{\rho} = 0.50/(0.50 + 23.0) = 0.02$ and the variance inflation factors by $C_1 = 3.725$ and $C_2 = 3.143$.

Thus the estimated standard error of $\bar{Y}_1 - \bar{Y}_2$ is given by

$$\widehat{SE}(\overline{Y}_1 - \overline{Y}_2) = S_P\left[\frac{C_1}{M_1} + \frac{C_2}{M_2}\right]^{1/2}$$

$$= 4.85\left[\frac{3.725}{1929} + \frac{3.143}{2205}\right]^{1/2} = 0.28$$

Therefore the adjusted $t$-statistic, with 30 degrees of freedom, is given by

$$t_A = \frac{\overline{Y}_1 - \overline{Y}_2}{\widehat{SE}(\overline{Y}_1 - \overline{Y}_2)}$$

$$= -\frac{0.36}{0.28} = -1.27 \quad (p = 0.21)$$

A 95 per cent confidence interval for $\mu_1 - \mu_2$, the mean difference in body mass index (kg/m$^2$), is given by $-0.36 \pm 2.042\,(0.28)$ or $(-0.93, 0.21)$.

*Further remarks*:

1. If $\rho$ is known, then an exact test of $H_0\colon \mu_1 = \mu_2$ may also be carried out using the individual as the unit of analysis. The appropriate $t$-test then has $M - 2$ degrees of freedom, where $M$ is the total number of individuals in the study (Blair and Higgins 1986). This suggests that an investigator may obtain considerable improvements in power by using external data to assign an *a priori* value to $\rho$. As pointed out by Murray (1997), this strategy could prove useful for analysing data from small trials as suitable estimates of intracluster correlation become increasingly available in the published literature. However, the potentially increased precision obtained from using an external estimate of $\rho$ must be weighed against the accompanying risk of bias resulting from a wrongly assessed value of this parameter. Given the sensitivity of statistical inferences to the assigned value of $\rho$, we would discourage this practice unless very reliable and representative external data are available.
2. Consistent with the comment in Section 6.2.1.3 regarding adjustment of the standard Pearson chi-square statistic, calculation of the adjusted $t$-statistic does not require that the pairwise correlation between any two observations in the same cluster is constant (e.g. Barcikowski 1981). In this case, $\hat{\rho}$ again measures the average degree of pairwise correlation, and the statistic $t_A$ remains valid (provided the assumption of a common variance $\sigma^2$ for the individual subject scores still holds).

**Mixed effects linear regression models**

An alternative approach for testing $H_0\colon \mu_1 = \mu_2$ is based on a two-stage nested analysis of variance model, a special case of the mixed effects linear regression model. This model, also referred to in some texts as a repeated measures analysis of variance model, is given by

$$Y_{ijl} = \mu + G_i + V_{ij} + e_{ijl} \qquad \begin{aligned} i &= 1,2 \\ j &= 1,2,\ldots,k_i \\ l &= 1,2,\ldots,m_{ij} \end{aligned} \tag{7.1}$$

The terms in this model include $\mu$, the true mean response (grand mean), and $G_i$, a constant representing the fixed effect of intervention group $i$ ($i = 1,2$) and constructed using dummy variables. Two random effects are also included in the model. Random cluster effects, denoted by $V_{ij}$, are assumed to be normally distributed with mean 0 and variance $\sigma_A^2$, i.e. $V_{ij} \sim N(0, \sigma_A^2)$. We similarly assume the error terms $e_{ijl} \sim N(0, \sigma_W^2)$.

Since the effects $G_i$ in equation (7.1) are considered fixed and the effects $V_{ij}$ random, the model in this equation may be described as mixed, with clusters regarded as nested within interventions, and subjects within clusters. The effects $V_{ij}$ and $e_{ijl}$ are assumed to be mutually independent, with the common intracluster correlation given by $\rho = \sigma_A^2/(\sigma_A^2 + \sigma_W^2)$, showing that this parameter measures the proportion of variance in $Y_{ijl}$ that can be attributed to the variation among clusters. If $\rho$ is

**Table 7.1** Analysis of variance corresponding to a completely randomized design in which $k$ clusters of size $m$ are assigned to each of two intervention groups

| Source of variation | Degrees of freedom | Sum of squares | Mean square | $F$ |
|---|---|---|---|---|
| Among intervention groups | 1 | SSG | MSG | MSG/MSC |
| Clusters within groups | $2(k-1)$ | SSC | MSC | |
| Subjects within clusters | $2k(m-1)$ | SSW | MSW | |

erroneously assumed to be zero, equivalent to omitting the terms $V_{ij}$ from the model, the resulting analysis will have an inflated type I error.

It would be a serious error to conduct the statistical analysis under equation (7.1) assuming the $V_{ij}$ are fixed, using, for example, dummy variables to represent cluster-to-cluster variation. Aside from the fact that the effect of each cluster in itself is not usually of interest, this strategy fails to disentangle the between-cluster variation from the effect of intervention (Zucker 1990, Rice and Leyland 1996). Thus even in the absence of a true intervention effect, a difference may appear to exist solely because of the differences between clusters assigned to the two groups. Consequently, the problem of inflated type I error remains.

A summary ANOVA table, which may be used to test the effect of intervention, i.e. to test $H_0: G_i = 0$, $i = 1, 2$, is shown in Table 7.1. The sources of variation and corresponding degrees of freedom, outlined in Table 7.1, are illustrated here for the case of $k$ clusters per intervention group and $m$ subjects per cluster. Note that the degrees of freedom for the appropriate error term in this table are given by $2(k-1)$, which depends only on the total number of clusters. This relatively small number of degrees of freedom may be regarded as a price to be paid for randomizing clusters rather than individuals.

The ANOVA outlined in Table 7.1 is strictly applicable to balanced designs only. An important advantage of such designs is that exact statistical inferences concerning the effect of intervention may be constructed. As noted in Section 6.1, the resulting test statistics are then identical to those obtained from cluster-level analyses (e.g. Koepsell *et al.* 1991). Of course, in practice the number of subjects per cluster may be highly variable. In this case, iterative approaches, such as generalized least squares, are usually the method of choice for fitting mixed effects linear regression models, since the associated procedures provide maximum likelihood estimates of the effect of intervention (Searle *et al.* 1992, Section 6.8). However, the resulting inferences, which may be obtained in practice using procedures such as PROC MIXED in the software package SAS, will now be approximate rather than exact (Dunn and Clark 1987, Ch. 6). Moreover, there is no unique method for calculating the degrees of freedom for this analysis (Littell *et al.* 1996, Ch. 2).

Equation (7.1) may also be rewritten to more clearly emphasize its interpretation as a regression model. This form of the equation may be written as

$$Y_{ijl} = \beta_0 + \beta_1 X_{ijl} + V_{ij} + e_{ijl}$$

where

$$X_{ijl} = \begin{cases} 1 & \text{if } i = 1 \text{ (experimental)} \\ 0 & \text{if } i = 2 \text{ (control)} \end{cases}$$

Using the SAS procedure PROC MIXED, the estimated effect of intervention in the worksite trial is given by $\hat{\beta}_1 = -0.36\,\text{kg/m}^2$, suggesting that subjects in the experimental group are slightly smaller in size than subjects in the control group. The approximate two-sample $t$-statistic with 30 degrees of freedom is given by

$$\begin{aligned} t_{\mathrm{M}} &= \hat{\beta}_1/\widehat{\mathrm{SE}}_{\mathrm{M}}(\hat{\beta}_1) \\ &= -0.36/0.30 = -1.23 \quad (p = 0.23) \end{aligned}$$

where $\widehat{\mathrm{SE}}_{\mathrm{M}}(\hat{\beta}_1)$ is the estimated standard error of $\hat{\beta}_1$. The accompanying 95 per cent confidence interval is given by $(-0.96, 0.24)$.

These results are analogous to those obtained using model-dependent GEE procedures that assume a working exchangeable correlation matrix. They may be computed, for example, using any GEE program capable of fitting linear regression models for correlated outcome data (e.g. the SAS procedure PROC GENMOD). An alternative approach is to calculate a robust variance estimator which avoids the model-dependent assumptions inherent in equation (7.1), but which also requires a larger number of clusters in each intervention group. For data arising from the worksite intervention trial, the results obtained are very similar, since the model-dependent and robust standard errors are both approximately equal to 0.30.

An interesting application of robust variance estimation is provided by Brook *et al.* (1983) in their analyses of the Rand Health Insurance Experiment (Newhouse and the Insurance Experimental Group 1993). In this study, approximately 2000 families from the United States were randomly assigned to one of 14 health insurance plans to evaluate the extent to which the provision of free care improves health. The analytic approach was based on a strategy suggested by Huber (1967), a special case of the more general procedure subsequently described by Liang and Zeger (1986). Further discussion of methods for obtaining robust variance estimators in the context of linear regression models is provided by Diggle *et al.* (1994, p. 69).

An alternative to classical analysis of variance or mixed effects linear regression is to apply a methodology often referred to in the behavioural science and educational literature as multilevel modelling (Goldstein 1995) or as hierarchical linear modelling (Bryk and Raudenbush 1992). A review of software available for multilevel modelling is given by Kreft *et al.* (1994).

Only recently have investigators recognized that there is a very close relationship among these approaches (see Raudenbush 1993, Ferron 1997, Singer 1998). For example, following Raudenbush (1993), the model in equation (7.1) may also be reexpressed as a multilevel model so that at the individual level (level I) we have

$$Y_{ijl} = \mu_{ij} + e_{ijl}, \qquad e_{ijl} \sim N(0, \sigma^2_{\mathrm{W}})$$

where $\mu_{ij}$ is the mean score for the $ij$th worksite. Furthermore, at the worksite level (level II), we may write

$$\mu_{ij} = \mu + G_i + V_{ij}, \qquad V_{ij} \sim N(0, \sigma^2_{\mathrm{A}})$$

While these simple algebraic equivalencies hold for linear regression models with quantitative outcome variables, they do not apply, in general, to the various extensions of logistic regression described in Chapter 6 (e.g. Neuhaus 1992). This is consistent with our observation at the beginning of Chapter 6 that the analytic issues involved in cluster randomization trials tend to be more complicated for binary than for quantitative outcome variables.

An extended form of the model in equation (7.1) may arise when repeated, independent cross-sectional samples of subjects are selected from each cluster over time. In this case, the main focus of interest is whether the trend over time in the mean level of $Y$ is significantly different in the two intervention groups. This question can be answered in the framework of a mixed model analysis of variance by focusing on the interaction between the effect of intervention and the secular effect of time. This extended model may be written as

$$Y_{ijlt} = \mu + G_i + T_t + V_{ij} + (GT)_{it} + (VT)_{jt(i)} + e_{ijlt} \qquad \begin{aligned} i &= 1,2 \\ j &= 1,2,\ldots,k_i \\ l &= 1,2,\ldots,m_{ij} \\ t &= 1,2,\ldots,T \end{aligned} \tag{7.2}$$

where the terms added to those in equation (7.1) include the fixed effects $T_t$, representing the secular effect of time in each group, the within-group interaction effects of time with the cluster effects $(VT)_{jt(i)}$, and the interaction effects of intervention with time $(GT)_{it}$. The intervention effect is tested by considering the statistical significance of the interaction term $(GT)_{it}$. This is done by comparing the source of variation attributable to this interaction to the mean square error for $(VT)_{jt(i)}$, which accounts for the possibility that the random effects $V_{ij}$ may not have identical distributions at each time point. Table 7.2 gives an outline of the corresponding ANOVA table for a balanced design. The appropriate error term for testing the effect of intervention is now seen to depend on the total number of time points as well as the number of clusters randomized.

Added to the assumptions underlying the simpler model given by equation (7.1) is the 'compound symmetry' assumption, which states for the extended model in equation (7.2) that the correlation between any two measurements over time on subjects from the same cluster is constant. As noted by several authors (e.g. Koepsell *et al.*1991), this assumption will often be violated in practice, although appropriate adjustments have been developed that may be usefully applied to data arising from individually randomized trials (e.g. Fleiss 1986, Section 8.1). Unfortunately, it is unclear whether such adjustments may be safely applied to cluster randomization trials, particularly when the cluster sizes are variable. Robust variance estimators may alternatively be adopted as a means of avoiding the fairly restrictive assumptions of compound symmetry (e.g. see Murray *et al.* 1998).

**Table 7.2** Analysis of variance corresponding to a completely randomized design in which $k$ clusters of size $m$ are assigned to each of two intervention groups with measurements taken on $T$ occasions

| Source of variation | Degrees of freedom | Sum of squares | Mean square | $F$ |
|---|---|---|---|---|
| Among intervention groups | 1 | SSG | MSG | |
| Time | $T-1$ | SST | MST | |
| Clusters within groups | $2(k-1)$ | SSC | MSC | |
| Intervention × time | $T-1$ | SSGT | MSGT | MSGT/MSCT |
| Clusters × time | $2(k-1)(T-1)$ | SSCT | MSCT | |
| Subjects within clusters | $2kT(m-1)$ | SSW | MSW | |

The model given in equation (7.2) corresponds to a cross-sectional design. Potentially greater power may be obtained when repeated assessments are made on the same subjects over time using a cohort design, since then the between-subject variation may be removed from the error term, as can be seen from an appropriately modified version of Table 7.2 (e.g. Koepsell *et al.* 1991, Feldman and McKinlay 1994). Nevertheless, as discussed above, it is technically preferable in the case of variable size clusters to construct inferences using likelihood-based procedures as implemented, for example, by PROC MIXED in SAS.

Gilliss *et al.* (1993) designed a cohort study to determine the efficacy of a psycho-educational nursing intervention in patients who received coronary artery bypass graft and valve repair surgery. As previously discussed in Section 3.2, a cluster randomization trial was planned in which the clusters consisted of consecutive groups of patients entered consecutively into the study. These temporal clusters were randomly assigned to one of two intervention groups, with quality-of-life measures collected at baseline, 4, 12 and 24 weeks. To test whether the resulting time pattern was the same in the two groups, a repeated measures ANOVA was used in which subjects were treated as random effects within clusters and clusters were treated as random effects within intervention groups. The intervention-by-time interaction provided a formal test of whether experimental group subjects improved more than control group subjects over the 24 weeks of the study.

A computationally simpler but algebraically equivalent alternative to repeated measures ANOVA occurs when measurements in a cohort study are taken at only two time points, including one at baseline ($T = 2$). In this case, one might choose to test the statistical significance of the difference in change scores from baseline in the two groups, an analysis which is easily understood and which provides a readily interpretable estimate of the intervention effect. An example of this approach is given by Walker *et al.* (1992).

## 7.1.2 Adjusting for covariates

For cohort designs when only two time points are involved, it was suggested in Section 7.1.1 that the analysis of difference scores (or change scores) may be an attractive strategy. However, there are potential drawbacks to this approach, since it involves assumptions that are not always realistic. One such assumption is that a unit increase in the baseline score is always associated with a unit increase in the final score or, equivalently, that the slope of the linear regression of the final score on the baseline score is 1.0. A violation of this assumption may lead to either an over- or under-adjustment of the post-intervention score (Murray *et al.* 1989). This problem may be avoided, at the loss of some simplicity in interpretation, by instead using the baseline score as a covariate in a mixed effects linear regression model. This approach has the flexibility of allowing the data to empirically determine the strength of the relationship between the baseline score and the final score, and then adjusting appropriately. As a result, covariate adjustment tends to be more powerful than an analysis based on change scores, particularly when the correlation between the baseline covariate and the response variable is weak. The regression approach also allows the intervention comparison to be adjusted for the influence of several baseline covariates simultaneously, measured at either the cluster or the individual level. As mentioned in Section 6.2.3, such adjustments can further increase the precision with which intervention effects are estimated, as well as account for chance imbalances on those variables that may distort the estimated effect of intervention. Such imbalances, if not controlled for at the design stage, can be adjusted for at the analysis stage through the use of a mixed effects linear regression model.

We illustrate adjustment for baseline scores using data from a cluster randomized trial of a counselling programme for the prevention of skin cancer (Mayer *et al.* 1998). A total of 54 pharmacies employing 178 pharmacists were randomized in equal numbers to receive either an educational programme for the prevention of skin cancer or a control intervention. Since random assignment of pharmacies was conducted separately within each of three national chains, a more precise analysis would account for the use of stratified randomization. We ignore this issue here for the purposes of illustration.

One of the principal study outcomes in this trial was a 12-item skin cancer knowledge test that was administered to all participating pharmacists at baseline and at a follow-up assessment. Scores ranged from 0 to 12, with 12 indicating complete accuracy. Analyses were limited to the subset of 101 pharmacists from 48 drugstores who provided all the requested data. This relatively low response rate may be a cause for concern, although the attrition rates are approximately the same in each group.

Suppose $k_i$ clusters are randomized to the $i$th group, $i = 1, 2$, with $m_{ij}$ individuals in each cluster, $j = 1, 2, \ldots, k_i$. We are interested in evaluating the effect of intervention after accounting for the influence of baseline knowledge score, age and sex. Letting $Y_{ijl}$ denote the knowledge score obtained at the follow-up assessment, the appropriate mixed effects linear regression model may be written as

$$Y_{ijl} = \beta_0 + \beta_1 X_{ijl} + \beta_2 Baseline_{ijl} + \beta_3 Age_{ijl} + \beta_4 Sex_{ijl} + V_{ij} + e_{ijl} \tag{7.3}$$

where

$$X_{ijl} = \begin{cases} 1 & \text{if } i = 1 \text{ (experimental)} \\ 0 & \text{if } i = 2 \text{ (control)} \end{cases}$$

and

$$Sex_{ijl} = \begin{cases} 1 & \text{if male} \\ 0 & \text{if female} \end{cases}$$

Baseline knowledge score is denoted in equation (7.3) by $Baseline_{ijl}$, age (in years) by $Age_{ijl}$ and sex by $Sex_{ijl}$. We also assume the random cluster effects $V_{ij} \sim N(0, \sigma_A^2)$, and the errors $e_{ijl} \sim N(0, \sigma_W^2)$. The intracluster correlation coefficient obtained after accounting for these covariates is then given by $\rho = \sigma_A^2/(\sigma_A^2 + \sigma_W^2)$.

In general, it is most worthwhile to adjust for those covariates which simultaneously influence outcome and have different distributions in the two intervention groups (Hauck *et al.* 1998). Nonetheless, covariate adjustment for a factor which is strongly related to outcome can improve precision even though it has the same distribution in both groups. Conversely, adjustment for a weakly correlated covariate may dilute statistical power and even compromise the validity of statistical inferences

**Table 7.3** Summary of analyses evaluating the effect of a skin cancer educational programme (Mayer *et al.* 1998)

| | Estimated regression coefficient | 95% confidence interval | Two-sided *p*-value |
|---|---|---|---|
| Effect of intervention (experimental vs. control) | 2.60 | (1.80, 3.40) | <0.01 |
| Baseline knowledge score | 0.47 | (0.30, 0.64) | <0.01 |
| Age (years) | 0.01 | (−0.04, 0.06) | 0.68 |
| Sex (male vs. female) | −0.85 | (−1.89, 0.19) | 0.11 |

when there are a limited number of clusters per intervention group. In this example, the baseline covariates defined above were fairly well balanced across intervention groups (see Mayer *et al.* 1998, Table 1).

Results obtained from fitting the model in equation (7.3) are provided in Table 7.3, where inferences were constructed using a robust variance estimator with a working exchangeable correlation matrix. After covariate adjustment, the average knowledge score among experimental group pharmacists was 2.6 points higher than among control group pharmacists. The corresponding 95 per cent confidence interval is given by $(1.80, 3.40)$.

An implicit assumption of the model in equation (7.3) is that the regression coefficients measuring the effects of the baseline variables are weighted averages of slopes calculated from cluster-level data (i.e. from an ecological analysis) and a common within-cluster slope (e.g. Scott and Holt 1982). The parameter being estimated is only interpretable when these slopes are approximately equal. However, differences between parameter estimates can be examined by comparing the results obtained when individual-level variables (e.g. age, sex) and their cluster-level versions (e.g. mean age, proportion male) are included in the same model, as previously discussed in Section 6.2.3.

## 7.2 The matched-pair design

### 7.2.1 Comparison of means

Let $d_j = \overline{Y}_{1j} - \overline{Y}_{2j}$ denote the mean difference in response between clusters in the $j$th pair (stratum), $j = 1, 2, \ldots, k$. Since there are only two clusters per stratum in the matched-pair design, estimates of between-cluster variability within a pair are totally confounded with the effect of intervention. Tests of the effect of intervention must therefore be calculated using between-stratum information on variability. One simple option is to apply the standard paired $t$-statistic to the mean differences $d_j = \overline{Y}_{1j} - \overline{Y}_{2j}$, $j = 1, 2, \ldots, k$, as computed between the clusters in a matched pair. Letting

$$\overline{d} = \sum_{j=1}^{k} \frac{d_j}{k} \quad \text{and} \quad S_d^2 = \sum_{j=1}^{k} \frac{(d_j - \overline{d})^2}{k-1}$$

denote the sample mean and variance, respectively, of the $d_j$, this statistic is given by $t_p = (\bar{d}\sqrt{k})/S_d$. An assumption underlying this test is that the $d_j$ are normally distributed about the same mean $\Delta$ with equal variances across strata. If these assumptions are satisfied, then the statistic $t_p$, with $k-1$ degrees of freedom, will provide an exact test of $H_0: \Delta = 0$. However, this test will usually be approximate as applied in practice, since cluster sizes tend to vary across strata (often through design), thus violating the assumption of equal variances. Violation of the normality assumption is not likely to be serious when $k$ is relatively large, since then the central limit theorem assures that $\bar{d}$ will have an approximate normal distribution even if outcomes for individual subjects are not normal.

A corresponding two-sided $(1-\alpha)100$ per cent confidence interval for $\Delta$ is given by $\bar{d} \pm t_{\alpha/2}S_d/\sqrt{k}$, where $t_{\alpha/2}$ is the $(1-\alpha)100$ per cent two-sided critical value of the $t$-distribution with $k-1$ degrees of freedom.

If relevant baseline information is available, the power of the paired $t$-test may be improved by computing the mean change from baseline for each cluster and replacing the $d_j$ by the difference in mean change for each pair of clusters. This approach was taken by Avorn *et al.* (1992), who studied six matched pairs of nursing homes. For one randomly selected nursing home in each pair, a group of trained health care workers provided the residents with an educational programme in geriatric psychopharmacology, with the other home in the pair serving as a control. Scores on an index of psychoactive drug use were taken both at baseline and 5 months after the intervention was administered. By using changes in these scores as the primary response variable, the investigators were able to show that the use of psychoactive drugs in nursing homes declined significantly more in those homes assigned to the experimental group.

In the presence of obvious non normality or gross heterogeneity in the variances of the $d_j$, reasonable alternatives to the paired $t$-test are the Wilcoxon signed rank test or Fisher's permutation test. These non-parametric procedures, discussed earlier in Section 6.3.1, assume that the differences $d_j$ are independently and symmetrically distributed, but impose no further distributional assumptions.

## 7.2.2 Adjusting for covariates

A pair-matching strategy can be used to control for the effect of known prognostic factors on outcome. However, there may be other factors influencing the response variable which are unknown in the design stage of a trial and which are not balanced between intervention groups. Therefore it may be necessary to adjust for such covariates in the analysis. Unfortunately, the difficulties involved in obtaining an estimate of between-cluster variability in a matched-pair design implies that direct adjustment may only be possible for those covariates measured at the cluster level (see Section 3.6). This can be done most conveniently by adapting an approach described by Rosner and Hennekens (1978) for the analysis of matched case–control and cohort studies. Consider the case of a single baseline covariate $X$ measured at the cluster level. Letting $d_j = \bar{Y}_{1j} - \bar{Y}_{2j}$ denote the difference in mean response between the clusters in a matched pair, this approach involves regressing $d_j$ on the difference $Z_j = \bar{X}_{1j} - \bar{X}_{2j}$, where $Z_j$ denotes the corresponding within-pair difference for the cluster-level covariate. For example, $Z_j$ might represent the difference in baseline smoking rates between two communities in a matched pair. Adjusted inferences for the effect of intervention may then be obtained by focusing on the estimated intercept of the resulting regression line. Since the true intercept is simply the expected value of the $d_j$ when $Z_j = 0$, comparing the estimated intercept to its standard error provides a test of whether the mean difference in response is statistically significant after adjusting for differences in $X$. This procedure is also easily extended to allow adjustment for several baseline covariates using multiple linear regression. The estimated intercept term in this regression may again be interpreted as the adjusted effect of intervention. Individual-level baseline covariates may also be adjusted for using this procedure, but only to the extent that they can be meaningfully modelled at the cluster level (see Section 6.3.3).

## *Example*

We illustrate methods for the analysis of quantitative data obtained from a matched-pair trial by analysing the cholesterol levels of men who participated in the British Family Heart Study (Family Heart Study Group 1994a). The purpose of the trial was to examine the effect of a 1-year, nurse-led lifestyle intervention on cardiovascular disease risk factors, with participating patients recruited from general medical practices.

Fifteen towns meeting specified demographic criteria were recruited for the study. Within each town, pairs of general medical practices with four to seven full-time partners each were invited to participate if they had similar patient populations and agreed to be randomized to either study arm. Male patients between the ages of 40 and 59 in these practices were considered eligible.

Mean serum cholesterol results obtained 1 year after randomization are shown in Table 7.4. For men in the control group, this was their first cholesterol evaluation, while men in the experimental group had their cholesterol levels taken at baseline as well. The securing of baseline measurements was in fact part of the experimental intervention, which included the identification of subjects at high risk for heart disease.

**Table 7.4** Mean serum cholesterol (mmol/l) levels for men in the British Family Heart Study at 1 year

| | Experimental | | | External control | | |
|---|---|---|---|---|---|---|
| Town | Number | Mean | SD | Number | Mean | SD |
| Portsmouth | 138 | 5.574 | 1.044 | 321 | 5.742 | 1.197 |
| Darlington | 156 | 5.812 | 1.235 | 335 | 5.831 | 1.048 |
| Gloucester | 173 | 5.651 | 1.188 | 176 | 5.714 | 1.204 |
| Carlisle | 180 | 5.438 | 0.965 | 345 | 6.067 | 1.401 |
| Burton | 142 | 5.595 | 0.979 | 257 | 5.702 | 1.365 |
| Lincoln | 116 | 5.530 | 0.931 | 249 | 5.717 | 1.206 |
| Dunfermline | 169 | 5.786 | 1.240 | 351 | 5.621 | 1.181 |
| Bridgend | 106 | 5.553 | 1.013 | 290 | 5.415 | 1.039 |
| Bury | 124 | 5.533 | 0.998 | 184 | 5.624 | 1.159 |
| Huddersfield | 147 | 5.594 | 1.115 | 215 | 5.752 | 1.030 |
| Ipswich | 120 | 5.391 | 0.916 | 285 | 5.585 | 1.050 |
| Newport | 75 | 5.629 | 1.107 | 263 | 5.619 | 1.122 |
| Poole | 118 | 5.370 | 0.903 | 242 | 5.515 | 1.076 |

SD, standard deviation.

**Table 7.5** Summary of test results obtained from a comparison of differences in mean serum cholesterol levels (mmol/l) in a matched-pair design

| Procedure | Test statistic | Two-sided *p*-value |
|---|---|---|
| Paired *t*-test | −2.07 (12 d.f.) | 0.06 |
| Wilcoxon signed rank test | Approximate | 0.04 |
| | Exact | 0.04 |
| Permutation test | Approximate | 0.06 |
| | Exact | 0.04 |

The following analysis begins by calculating a difference in mean cholesterol levels for men in the experimental and control group practices. The mean of these differences may be obtained as −0.11 with standard error 0.05, indicating that the intervention resulted in only a modest reduction in cholesterol level. The two-sided paired *t*-statistic for testing the null hypothesis that the true mean difference is equal to zero is given by −2.07 ($p = 0.06$, 12 df), with 95 per cent confidence limits given by $(-0.23, 0.01)$. A similar result was obtained by Thompson *et al.* (1997b, Table 4) who accounted for between-cluster variability using a maximum likelihood approach. However, their approach also took into account the variability in cluster size that is ignored by the *t*-test.

It is interesting to note that exact inferences constructed using either the Wilcoxon signed rank test ($p = 0.04$) or an exact permutation test ($p = 0.04$) are statistically significant, with both analyses carried out using the software package Proc-StatXact (Mehta and Patel 1997). The observed discrepancies between the different statistical procedures, as summarized in Table 7.5, may be a consequence of results observed in the town of Carlisle, which experienced an average difference in mean cholesterol levels more than twice that of any other community (Thompson *et al.* 1997b).

We conclude this example by noting that the number of subjects who received the intervention in each practice was consistently smaller than the number of subjects in the corresponding control group practice. This imbalance occurred partly because half the men attending the experimental group practices were randomly assigned to an internal control group, and partly because of systematic oversampling of subjects from the control group practices. The final imbalance in sample sizes may also reflect the resistance to repeated assessment among men who were assigned the lifestyle intervention.

Gail *et al.* (1996) review the effect of planned imbalance across intervention groups on the validity of *t*-tests and permutation tests. Their results suggest that the properties of these tests will not be seriously disturbed unless the analyses are performed on fewer than six matched pairs.

## 7.3 The stratified design

The analyses for a stratified cluster randomization design may be based on straightforward extensions of methods described in Section 7.1 for the analyses of data obtained from a completely randomized design. Such extensions are natural because the stratified design may be viewed as a replication of the completely randomized design in each of the S strata.

For purposes of illustration, we limit attention to a design allocating $n_j$ clusters to each intervention group within stratum $j$, with $m_j$ subjects per cluster in the $j$th stratum, $j = 1, 2, \ldots, S$. We further assume that the trial gives rise to the stratum-specific intervention effects measured by $d_j = \overline{Y}_{1j} - \overline{Y}_{2j}$, $j = 1, 2, \ldots, S$. Each $d_j$ is assumed to estimate the true mean difference in response $\Delta$, with

$$\mathrm{Var}(d_j) = \frac{2\sigma^2}{m_j n_j}[1 + (m_j - 1)\rho]$$

i.e. it is assumed there is no intervention by stratum interaction. Our aim is to test the null hypothesis $H_0{:}\, \Delta = 0$.

Following the approach described by Schwartz *et al.* (1980, pp. 190–191), the appropriate test statistic may be based on the weighted mean difference

$$\overline{d}_W = \frac{\sum_{j=1}^{S} W_j d_j}{\sum_{j=1}^{S} W_j}$$

with the weights $W_j$ chosen to reflect the relative amount of information in the $d_j$. From the definition of $\overline{d}_W$, we have

$$\widehat{\mathrm{Var}}(\overline{d}_W) = \frac{\sum_{j=1}^{S} W_j^2\, \widehat{\mathrm{Var}}(d_j)}{\left(\sum_{j=1}^{S} W_j\right)^2}$$

where $\widehat{\mathrm{Var}}(d_j)$ estimates $\mathrm{Var}(d_j)$ obtained by replacing $\sigma^2$ and $\rho$ by pooled estimates of these parameters calculated over the $S$ strata. The weights $W_j$ may then be taken as the reciprocals of the $\widehat{\mathrm{Var}}(d_j)$.

The resulting test statistic $t = \overline{d}_W / [\widehat{\mathrm{Var}}(\overline{d}_W)]^{1/2}$ may be regarded as an approximate $t$-statistic with $2\sum_{j=1}^{S}(n_j - 1) = K - 2S$ degrees of freedom under $H_0{:}\, \Delta = 0$, where $K$ is the total number of clusters randomized. An approximate $(1 - \alpha)100$ per cent confidence interval about $\Delta$ may be similarly computed as $\overline{d}_W \pm t_{\alpha/2}[\widehat{\mathrm{Var}}(\overline{d}_W)]^{1/2}$, where $t_{\alpha/2}$ is the $(1 - \alpha)100$ per cent two-sided critical value of the $t$-distribution with $K - 2S$ degrees of freedom.

If the cluster sizes vary within a given combination of intervention and stratum, the $\mathrm{Var}(d_j)$ in the development above may be replaced by

$$\sigma^2\left[\frac{C_{1j}}{M_{1j}} + \frac{C_{2j}}{M_{2j}}\right]$$

where $M_{ij}$ denotes the total number of individuals receiving intervention $i$ in stratum $j$, and the $C_{ij}$, $i = 1, 2$, are defined as in Section 6.4.

Individual-level analyses for this design may also be conducted using a mixed effects linear regression model similar to the model presented in equation (7.1), but adding indicator variables to represent the differences among strata. Alternatively, exact cluster-level analyses may be performed using non-parametric procedures, as described in Section 6.4.

# 8

# Analysis of count, time to event and categorical outcomes

The primary outcome variable in most cluster randomization trials is either binary or continuous. However, this is not always the case. We therefore focus in the following sections on the statistical analysis of count, time to event and categorical data, each of which has been of interest in a number of cluster randomization trials. For example, Payment *et al.* (1991), in a study involving count data, examined the effect of a domestic water filter on reducing gastrointestinal symptomatology. Participating households were randomly assigned either to receive a domestic water filter or to continue using their usual source of drinking water. The annual number of gastro-intestinal episodes was determined for each household member in order to assess the effect of intervention. However, standard methods for the analysis of count data (e.g. Breslow and Day 1987) were correctly recognized as being inappropriate, since each episode would then be counted as an independent event. Methods which allowed for correlation in the number of episodes per household were adopted instead.

Morris *et al.* (1994), in a trial involving time to event data, revisited data from a study in which 18 of 36 nursing homes were randomly assigned to receive an intervention consisting of higher per diem payments, as well as bonuses for discharging patients within 90 days. Thus a primary goal of the trial was to evaluate the effectiveness of the intervention in reducing length of stay. However, approximately 20 per cent of the 1601 study subjects were not yet discharged from the participating nursing homes by the end of the study. Using standard clinical trial terminology, these observations are said to be truncated or censored, raising special analytic challenges (Kleinbaum 1996). However, the standard methods used for accounting for censoring assume that the times to event are statistically independent. Therefore, these methods are not directly applicable to cluster randomization trials. More appropriate methods for both time to event and count data are presented in Section 8.1, separately by study design. Section 8.2 deals with statistical issues raised by the need to analyse ordinal or nominal outcome variables.

# 8.1 Count and time to event data

## 8.1.1 The completely randomized design

### *8.1.1.1 Standard methods of analysis*

If subjects are followed for varying lengths of times, it is clear that crude event rates or simple proportions are not an appropriate measure of the success of an intervention. An alternative approach frequently adopted in many clinical trials is to ascertain the number of events that occur relative to the total follow-up time, yielding an incidence rate that accounts for the variable follow-up.

Consider, for example, a trial comparing treatments for children with otitis media, defined as inflammation of the middle ear (Le and Lindgren 1996). Ventilation tubes were surgically placed in both of a child's ears to prevent any further hearing impairment and to reduce the frequency of future episodes of otitis media. Since any benefits that can be attributed to the presence of these tubes are only available while they remain unblocked and in place, the primary outcome variable in this trial was the time to tube failure. Following surgery, children were randomly assigned either to receive prednisone and sulfamethoprim treatment for 2 weeks or to receive a control treatment. A factor complicating the analysis was that children randomized earlier in the 3-year accrual period were more likely to have a longer length of follow-up than children randomized towards the end of the trial.

Clusters are defined in this study as the set of paired times to tube failure provided by each child. Although in previous chapters we have focused almost exclusively on trials in which the cluster was composed of different individuals, similar analytic challenges arise in trials for which multiple outcomes are available on each study subject. Methods that account for the effects of this form of clustering have been extensively discussed in the ophthalmological literature, where data may be obtained from either one or two eyes (e.g. Ederer 1973, Glynn and Rosner 1992). Similar discussion has also appeared in the dental literature (e.g. Imrey 1986, Imrey and Chilton 1992), in studies of coronary artery bypass, where each subject may have one or more grafts (Henderson *et al.* 1988), in orthopaedics, where multiple degenerative joints are assessed for each patient (Morris 1993), and in studies where data are available from one or both ears of each subject (e.g. Coren and Hakstian 1990).

The primary aim of the otitis media trial was to compare the rate of tube failure across intervention groups. This goal may be formalized by establishing the null hypothesis $H_0$: $\lambda_1 = \lambda_2$, where $\lambda_1$ and $\lambda_2$ are the underlying rates of tube failure in the experimental and control groups, respectively. Suppose that $k_i$ clusters (children) are randomized to intervention group $i, i = 1, 2$, with $Y_{ijl}$ denoting the response of the $l$th cluster member (ear) in the $j$th cluster of group $i$, where $Y_{ijl} = 1$ if tube failure has occurred by time $t_{ijl}$ and $Y_{ijl} = 0$ otherwise. Then $Y_{ij} = \sum_{l=1}^{2} Y_{ijl}$ and $t_{ij} = \sum_{l=1}^{2} t_{ijl}$, respectively, denote the total number of failures and the total follow-up time in the $ij$th cluster, $j = 1, \ldots, k_i$. Using a notation similar to that in Chapter 6, we denote the observed cluster-specific incidence rates by $\hat{\lambda}_{ij} = Y_{ij}/t_{ij}$. Then the observed incidence rate for the $i$th intervention group is given by $\hat{\lambda}_i = Y_i/t_i$ where $Y_i = \sum_{j=1}^{k_i} Y_{ij}$ and $t_i = \sum_{j=1}^{k_i} t_{ij}$.

**Table 8.1** Summary data from a randomized trial evaluating the effect of ventilating tubes placed in ears of children with otitis media (Le and Lindgren 1996)

| Characteristic | Intervention group | |
|---|---|---|
| | Surgery plus predisone and sulfamethoprim (experimental) | Surgery alone (control) |
| Number of children | 40 | 38 |
| Cluster size | 2 | 2 |
| Number of tubes implanted | 80 | 76 |
| Number of tubes failed | 75 | 69 |
| Time until tubes failed (ear-months) | 806.8 | 567 |
| Rate of failure (failures/ear-month) | 0.09 | 0.12 |

Table 8.1 summarizes the failure time data arising from this trial. Of the 80 tubes placed in the ears of 40 children randomly assigned to the experimental group, $Y_1 = 75$ failed over the $t_1 = 806.8$ ear-months during which data were collected. Similarly $Y_2 = 69$ of the 76 tubes placed in the ears of 38 children in the control group failed over $t_2 = 567.0$ ear-months of follow-up. The observed failure rates for the two groups are then given, respectively, by

$$\begin{aligned}\hat{\lambda}_1 &= Y_1/t_1 \\ &= 75/806.8 \\ &= 0.093 \text{ tubes per ear-month}\end{aligned}$$

and

$$\begin{aligned}\hat{\lambda}_2 &= Y_2/t_2 \\ &= 69/567.0 \\ &= 0.122 \text{ tubes per ear-month}\end{aligned}$$

Thus the observed rate ratio comparing the tube failure rates in the two groups can be computed as

$$\begin{aligned}\widehat{RR} &= \hat{\lambda}_1/\hat{\lambda}_2 \\ &= 0.093/0.122 \\ &= 0.76\end{aligned}$$

Suppose there is no between-cluster variation in the rate of tube failure, or, equivalently, that the times to tube failure for the right and left ears of a child are uncorrelated. Then inferences concerning the rate ratio parameter $\widehat{RR} = \lambda_1/\lambda_2$ may be constructed by assuming that the number $Y_i$ of tubes which fail in the $i$th intervention group follows a Poisson distribution with true failure rate $\lambda_i$, $i = 1, 2$, during the $t_i$ ear-months of follow-up. In this case, the estimated variance of $\ln(\widehat{RR})$ is given (Rosner 1995, p. 593) by $(1/Y_1) + (1/Y_2)$. It therefore follows that an approximate one degree of freedom chi-square test of $H_0$: $RR = 1$ is obtained using the statistic

$$\chi^2_{RR} = \frac{[\ln(\widehat{RR}) - 0]^2}{(1/Y_1) + (1/Y_2)}$$

$$= \frac{[\ln(0.76)]^2}{(1/75) + (1/69)} = 2.61 \quad (p = 0.11)$$

The associated 95 per cent confidence interval for $RR$ is then given by

$$\left(e^{\ln(0.76) - [1.96\sqrt{(1/75) + (1/69)}]}, e^{\ln(0.76) + [1.96\sqrt{(1/75) + (1/69)}]}\right)$$

or $(0.55, 1.06)$. It cannot therefore be concluded with 95 per cent confidence that the true value of $RR$ is different from 1.

The analysis described above focuses on the comparison of tube failure rates. Suppose the primary endpoint in this trial were defined instead to be the time in months until tube failure. Assuming the Poisson assumption described above is valid, equivalent inferences would be obtained if the time to failure of the $l$th tube, $l = 1, 2$, from the $j$th child, $j = 1, \ldots, k_i$ in the $i$th intervention group were assumed independently to follow an exponential distribution with mean $1/\lambda_i$. This equivalence is intuitively sensible, since if the rate of tube failure is high, the corresponding mean time to tube failure should be correspondingly short. Further discussion of the close relationship between the Poisson distribution and the exponential distribution is given from a non-technical perspective by Flanders and Kleinbaum (1995).

Unfortunately statistical inferences which assume that the number of events per intervention group follows a Poisson distribution are not appropriate for cluster randomization trials. This is because the presence of between-cluster variation in event rates or, equivalently, of correlated failure times, inflates the variance of the observed rate ratio. We will therefore explore three different analytic approaches for constructing inferences concerning the effect of intervention in this case. These include (1) cluster-level analyses, (2) procedures based on extensions of the Poisson distribution which allow for between-cluster variability (i.e. procedures for over-dispersed Poisson data), and (3) suitable adjustments of the Cox proportional hazards model. These methods are illustrated using data from the otitis media trial where there are two members per cluster, but are also applicable to cluster randomization trials involving a variable number of subjects per cluster.

It is important to note that we deliberately omit any consideration of adjustments to standard statistical procedures based on the calculation of a simple variance inflation factor. For quantitative and binary outcome data, this term is given by $1 + (m - 1)\rho$, where $m$ denotes the number of individuals per cluster and $\rho$ the value of intracluster correlation. In Chapter 6 we described how variance inflation factors of this form may be used to adjust standard procedures such as the Pearson chi-square test for the effect of clustering. Unfortunately, difficulties in finding appropriate measures of intracluster correlation have prevented derivation of parallel adjustments for overdispersed Poisson data or for correlated survival data (see Segal *et al.* 1997).

Our discussion of count and time to event data is limited primarily to studies where a cohort of subjects is identified from each cluster prior to random assignment and then followed until the end of the trial. Time on study may then vary among subjects.

However, count data are also of interest in trials enrolling samples of subjects selected independently at one or more cross-sectional surveys. Time on study is then no longer relevant. For example, the number of cigarettes each student smokes in the week prior to being surveyed might be of interest in school-based smoking prevention trials (e.g. Siddiqui *et al.* 1999). Methods of analysis described in Section 8.1.1.3, as based on either the mixed-effects Poisson regression model or the generalized estimating equations approach, are also applicable in this context.

### 8.1.1.2 Cluster-level analyses

The simplest statistical approach is to conduct the analysis at the cluster level, using the observed rate of tube failure per ear-month for each child as a summary measure, where this rate is defined as $\hat{\lambda}_{ij} = Y_{ij}/t_{ij}$. This leads to a straightforward comparison of the mean rates of failure $\overline{\lambda}_1$ and $\overline{\lambda}_2$, where $\overline{\lambda}_i = \sum_{j=1}^{k_i} \hat{\lambda}_{ij}/k_i$. Although this comparison provides a natural method of evaluating the effect of intervention, other summary statistics may sometimes be of greater interest. For example, Ray *et al.* (1997), in their trial of a consultation service intended to reduce falls among nursing home residents, estimated the proportion of residents who fell more than twice in a year by constructing Kaplan–Meier (product-limit) survival curves. This trial will be discussed further in Section 8.1.2.

We now revisit the otitis media trial introduced in Section 8.1.1.1. For these data, it may be calculated that $\overline{\lambda}_1 = 0.13$ with corresponding standard deviation given by 0.11. A much larger mean rate of failure, given by $\overline{\lambda}_2 = 0.21$ (standard deviation 0.29), may be calculated for children in the control group. The difference in mean failure rates between children in the two groups is consequently equal to $\overline{\lambda}_1 - \overline{\lambda}_2 = -0.08$. Using a two sample $t$-test with 76 degrees of freedom, the two-sided $p$-value is then obtained as 0.09. We also note that similar results are obtained using either a permutation test or the Wilcoxon rank sum test, as may be computed using the software package Proc-StatXact (Mehta and Patel 1997).

The analysis described above has several limitations. For example, all cluster-specific estimates of the tube failure rates $\hat{\lambda}_{ij}$ are regarded as equally precise, an assumption which is not usually reasonable in practice. Thus, if the number of tube failures follows a Poisson distribution, the estimated variance of $\hat{\lambda}_{ij}$ is given by $\hat{\lambda}_{ij}/t_{ij}$, a function of both time on study and the observed failure rate (Flanders and Kleinbaum 1995). This suggests that individual-level analyses, such as those discussed in Sections 8.1.1.3 and 8.1.1.4, may be preferable.

### 8.1.1.3 Extensions of Poisson regression

**Ratio estimator approach**

Statistical inferences for the observed rate ratio $\widehat{RR}$ can also be derived using the theory of ratio estimation. This theory, used by Rao and Scott (1992) for developing an analytic approach to the analysis of correlated binary data, also underlies the generalized estimating equations approach (see Lavange *et al.* 1994). It follows from this theory that the estimated variance of the observed failure rate for the $i$th intervention group is given by (Ahn and Lee 1997, Rao and Scott 1999)

$$\widehat{\text{Var}}(\hat{\lambda}_i) = \frac{k_i}{k_i - 1} \sum_{j=1}^{k_i} \frac{t_{ij}^2}{t_i^2} (\hat{\lambda}_{ij} - \hat{\lambda}_i)^2$$

The variance of $\ln(\widehat{RR})$ may then be estimated by

$$\widehat{\text{Var}}[\ln(\widehat{RR})] = \frac{\widehat{\text{Var}}(\hat{\lambda}_1)}{\hat{\lambda}_1^2} + \frac{\widehat{\text{Var}}(\hat{\lambda}_2)}{\hat{\lambda}_2^2} \tag{8.1}$$

which may be computed for the otitis media data as 0.0164.

An approximate one degree of freedom chi-square test of $H_0$: $RR = 1$ is then given by the statistic

$$\begin{aligned}\chi^2_{\text{RB}} &= \frac{[\ln(\widehat{RR}) - 0]^2}{\widehat{\text{Var}}[\ln(\widehat{RR})]} \\ &= \frac{[\ln(0.76)]^2}{0.0164} \\ &= 4.42 \quad (p = 0.03)\end{aligned}$$

The associated 95 per cent confidence interval for $\widehat{RR}$ can now be computed as

$$\left(e^{\ln(0.76) - [1.96\sqrt{0.0164}]}, e^{\ln(0.76) + [1.96\sqrt{0.0164}]}\right)$$

or $(0.60, 0.98)$.

Since this confidence interval excludes 1.0, we might conclude that the intervention has reduced the tube failure rate. One possible explanation for this result, which is inconsistent with that found in our earlier analyses, may be related to the underlying assumption that the rate of tube failure is constant throughout the study. Since violation of this assumption is known to produce aberrant results (see Vaeth 1979), we explore this issue further in Section 8.1.1.4 by presenting a less restrictive analysis.

**Parametric models**

Parametric models for the analysis of overdispered count data or correlated survival data have not been widely used. For those studies which have adopted a fully parametric approach, perhaps the most popular model has been based on the assumption of an underlying negative binomial distribution. This distribution results when (i) the number of events within a cluster follows a Poisson distribution conditional on the rate parameters $\lambda_{ij}$ and $t_{ij}$; and (ii) the cluster-specific tube failure rates $\lambda_{ij}$ are assumed to vary across cluster sizes in accordance with a gamma distribution (Gardner *et al.* 1995). The negative binomial distribution also arises as a special case of the beta-binomial distribution when cluster sizes are large and the overall tube failure rate is small.

Regression models based on the negative binomial distribution can be fitted using a procedure available in the statistical package Stata (StataCorp 1997), with parameter estimates obtained using the method of maximum likelihood. A one degree of freedom likelihood ratio test of $H_0$: $RR = 1$ then gives $\chi^2_{\text{N}} = 2.59$ ($p = 0.11$). As with the beta-binomial distribution, a two degree of freedom test can also be constructed. For count data this would provide a test sensitive to the effect of intervention on either the tube failure rate or the degree of overdispersion. We omit further consideration of such a procedure here, since it tends not to be of great practical interest.

An alternative model for overdispersed Poisson data assumes that the log transform of the expected number of tube failures follows a normal distribution across clusters (Goldstein 1995, pp. 106–108). This mixed-effects Poisson regression model is analogous to the logistic-normal model previously discussed in Chapter 6. Although variables measured at either the cluster or the individual level may be included in this model, an important practical limitation is that estimated effects of intervention may be difficult to interpret (Segal *et al.* 1997).

**Generalized estimating equations approach**

Investigators seldom have sufficient information to validate the assumption that the cluster-specific tube failure rates follow a specific parametric distribution (e.g. gamma). Thus approaches which make fewer assumptions are often preferred in practice. One such approach, suitable for overdispersed count data, is based on a weighted version of Poisson regression (Breslow 1984). However, since the required weights would generally be defined as the reciprocal of the variance of the number of events per cluster, it is clear that the variance of $Y_{ij}$ must be specified. This approach, which is the Poisson analogue of the approach proposed by Williams (1982) for the analysis of correlated binary data, was adopted by Sommer *et al.* (1986) in their trial examining the effect of vitamin A supplementation on childhood mortality. A limitation of both procedures is that adjustment is restricted to variables measured at the cluster level. Furthermore, the validity of inferences constructed with these procedures depends on the correct specification of the imposed weights, i.e. inferences are based on a special case of GEE using model-based variance estimators.

These problems were addressed by Segal and Neuhaus (1993), who exploited the relationship between count data and time to event data. As noted above, if the number of events within a specified time interval follows a Poisson distribution, then the time between events necessarily follows an exponential distribution. This relationship allows Poisson regression procedures (e.g. the SAS procedure PROC GENMOD SAS, Institute. Inc. 1997) to be used for the analysis of exponential survival data. The robust variance estimator popularized by Liang and Zeger (1986) can then be used to account for the effects of clustering. Provided the number of clusters is large, the precision with which the regression coefficients are estimated can be improved by fitting a weighted Poisson regression model. The estimated coefficients will then be identical to those described by Breslow (1984), assuming all covariates are measured at the cluster level. However, for simplicity, we limit our attention to models which do not incorporate such weights. In the context of the estimating equations literature, this is known as using an independent working correlation matrix.

The estimated regression coefficient for the effect of intervention is now algebraically identical to $\ln(\widehat{RR}) = \ln(\hat{\lambda}_1/\hat{\lambda}_2)$, with estimated variance obtained using equation (8.1). We also note that the variance estimator available in the SAS procedure PROC GENMOD differs only in omitting the terms $k_i/(k_i - 1)$ (Lavange *et al.* 1994).

Aberrant results obtained using Poisson regression models could be a consequence of the implicit assumption that there is a fixed rate of tube failure. In the context of time to event data, this is equivalent to assuming a fixed hazard rate. However, this assumption can be relaxed using the Cox proportional hazards model, as discussed in the following section.

### *8.1.1.4 Extensions of the Cox proportional hazards model*

An indicated above, an appealing feature of Cox proportional hazards regression as compared with Poisson regression is that it does not require the assumption of a fixed rate of tube failure over time. The possibly varying rate of tube failure over time is known as the hazard function $h(t)$. Denoting the experimental and control groups by $i = 1, 2$, respectively, the effect of intervention may be tested using a Cox regression model given by

$$h(t|X_{ijl}) = h_0(t)\exp(X_{ijl}\beta) \qquad (8.2)$$

where

$$X_{ijl} = \begin{cases} 1 & \text{if } i = 1 \\ 0 & \text{if } i = 2 \end{cases}$$

for the $l$th ear, $l = 1, 2$, of the $j$th child, $j = 1, 2, \ldots k_i$. The term $h_0(t)$ in equation (8.2) denotes the baseline hazard reflecting the (possibly time-varying) tube failure rate for children in the control group. Thus the hazard function for children in the $i$th group is given by

$$h(t|X_{1jl}) = h_0(t)\exp(\beta) \qquad \text{if } i = 1$$

and

$$h(t|X_{2jl}) = h_0(t) \qquad \text{if } i = 2$$

The effect of intervention is then given by the hazard ratio

$$\begin{aligned} HR &= h(t|X_{1jl})/h(t|X_{2jl}) \\ &= \exp(\beta) \end{aligned}$$

This expression shows that the effect of intervention is to multiply the possibly time-varying baseline hazard by the parameter $HR = \exp(\beta)$, assumed to be fixed over time. This relationship between the hazard functions for children in the control and experimental groups is a key assumption of the Cox model, explaining why it is referred to as a proportional hazards model. An introduction to the Cox model is provided by Rosner (1995, Section 13.9), while more advanced discussion is provided by Hosmer and Lemeshow (1999) and Kleinbaum (1996).

It is interesting to note that rate ratios obtained from a Poisson regression model may also be interpreted as hazard ratios. Furthermore, the results obtained from fitting a Poisson regression model will be similar to those obtained using a Cox model when the hazard rate is fixed over time.

Statistical inferences obtained using Cox regression typically assume that the survival times are independent. For the otitis media trial, this independence assumption is unlikely to hold since the tube failure times for the two ears belonging to the same subject will almost certainly be correlated. We will therefore consider extensions of the standard Cox model that relax this assumption. It should also be noted that similar assumptions of independence are required for closely related methods such as the logrank test (Rosner 1995, Section 13.8), thus also prohibiting their use in the present context.

Several extensions of the Cox model that account for the effects of clustering have been developed. Approaches that are particularly relevant to the analysis of data arising from cluster randomization trials can be based on either frailty models or marginal models (Segal *et al.* 1997). Frailty models account for the effects of clustering by allowing the hazard function to vary at random among clusters. These models are analogous to mixed-effects logistic regression models commonly used for the analysis of correlated binary outcome data. However, since estimates of the effect of intervention may be difficult to interpret with frailty models, we focus here on marginal models instead. These models are convenient in that they allow inferences to be constructed by first using a standard Cox regression analysis to obtain point estimates of the effect of intervention. The effects of clustering are then accounted for by using a robust variance estimator based on extensions of the approach popularized by Liang and Zeger (1986). The resulting model is attractive in that it may include variables measured at either the cluster level, including intervention status, or the individual level (e.g. age, sex). However, available evidence suggests that inferences based on robust variance estimators require at least 20 clusters in each intervention group in order to ensure their validity (e.g. Lin 1994).

We illustrate these methods using data from the otitis media trial. The estimated hazard ratio of tube failure may be computed using standard Cox regression as $\widehat{HR} = 0.70$, which suggests that the intervention lowers the risk of tube failure. Denoting the robust variance estimator of $\hat{\beta} = \ln(\widehat{HR})$ by $\widehat{\text{Var}}_{\text{CR}}(\hat{\beta})$, an approximate one degree of freedom chi-square test of $H_0$: $HR = 1$ is then given by the statistic

$$\chi^2_{\text{CR}} = \frac{(\hat{\beta} - 0)^2}{\widehat{\text{Var}}_{\text{CR}}(\hat{\beta})} = \frac{[\ln(0.70)]^2}{0.035} = 3.55 \quad (p = 0.06)$$

The corresponding 95 per cent confidence interval for $HR$ may then be computed as

$$(\mathrm{e}^{\ln(0.70) - [1.96\sqrt{0.035}]}, \mathrm{e}^{\ln(0.70) + [1.96\sqrt{0.035}]})$$

or $(0.49, 1.01)$.

We also note that application of the Cox model using standard variance estimators would have resulted in (spurious) statistical significance. Similar conclusions were reached by Le and Lindgren (1996).

The analyses above were conducted using robust variance estimators for the Cox model provided by the statistical package Stata (StataCorp 1997). However, these variances may also be obtained using the statistical package SUDAAN (Shah *et al.* 1996) or by applying SAS macros (Lin 1994). Results of all the analyses considered in Section 8.1.1 are summarized in Table 8.2.

It is very common to supplement inferences concerning time to event data by plotting Kaplan–Meier (product-limit) survival curves (e.g. Rosner 1995, Section 13.7). These curves, which estimate the probability of surviving beyond time $t$, may fortunately be constructed as if all survival times were independent (Ying and Wei 1994). However, standard methods for obtaining corresponding variance estimators, using, for example, Greenwood's formula (Hosmer and Lemeshow 1999, Section 2.3), are not appropriate and will result in biased statistical inferences (e.g. Williams 1995).

Figure 8.1 provides Kaplan–Meier survival curves for time to tube failure by intervention group. These curves estimate the average tube survival probability across

**Table 8.2** Summary of analyses evaluating the effect of ventilating tubes placed in the ears of children with otitis media (Le and Lindgren 1996)

| Procedure | Estimated hazard ratio | 95 per cent confidence interval | Two-sided *p*-value |
|---|---|---|---|
| Two-sample *t*-test | – | – | 0.09 |
| Permutation test | | | |
| Approximate | – | – | 0.09 |
| Exact | – | – | 0.09 |
| Poisson regression | 0.76 | (0.55, 1.06) | 0.11 |
| Poisson regression adjusted for clustering (GEE robust) | 0.76 | (0.60, 0.98) | 0.03 |
| Proportional hazards regression | 0.70 | (0.50, 0.98) | 0.04 |
| Proportional hazards regression adjusted for clustering | 0.70 | (0.49, 1.01) | 0.06 |

clusters within an intervention group (Aalen *et al.* 1995). Since all tubes were viable at study entry, the survival curves yield a probability of 1.0 at time $t = 0$ months. The curves will only fall when a tube fails, resulting in an observed step function. The size of the step will reflect the number of tubes which fail at a specified time, as well as the number of tubes still functioning. Note that the survival curve for

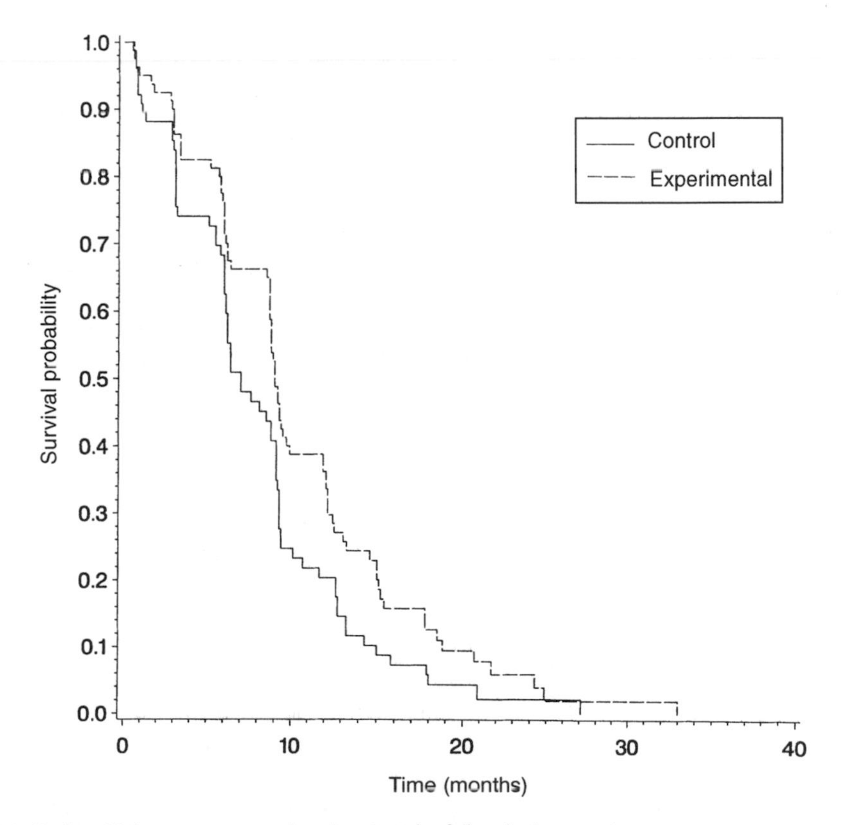


**Fig. 8.1** Kaplan–Meier curves comparing time to tube failure by intervention group.

children in the experimental group is always greater than that for children in the control group, implying that the intervention has increased tube survival time. From our analyses using the Cox model, the observed benefits of the experimental intervention are seen not to be statistically significant.

## 8.1.2 Matched-pair and stratified designs

We now discuss analyses for count or time to event data as obtained from matched-pair and stratified cluster randomization trials. If there are a sufficient number of clusters in each stratum and intervention group, the regression models described in Section 8.1.1 may be safely used for stratified designs, and therefore no new methodology is required. We therefore focus most of our attention in this section on matched-pair designs.

Analyses for matched-pair trials may be illustrated using data reported by Ray *et al.* (1997) from a randomized trial of a consultation service developed to help prevent falls and associated injuries in high-risk nursing home residents. Seven pairs of nursing homes were enrolled, matched by geographic proximity and the number of available beds.

Time on study began when the programme assessments were initiated in the nursing homes assigned to the intervention group, thus further matching the homes for calendar time. Study subjects were followed for up to 1 year after the index date, with observations censored for various reasons, including death or discharge.

The effect of intervention was assessed using two primary endpoints, the mean proportion of recurrent fallers in 1 year and the incidence rate of injurious falls (per 100 person-years). The proportion of recurrent fallers (defined as a resident having two or more falls during follow-up) could not be directly calculated since not all residents were followed for the same length of time. Instead, separate Kaplan–Meier curves were constructed for each nursing home. These curves were used to obtain the proportion of recurrent fallers during the 1 year follow-up. Falls requiring medical treatment (e.g. hospitalization, emergency department visit, physician visit or on-site radiological examination) were defined to be injurious. The rate of injurious falls was calculated as the number of injurious falls divided by the person-years of follow-up.

Summary data provided in Table 8.3 show that the mean percentage of recurrent fallers is equal to 43.7 per cent in the intervention facilities as compared with 54.1 per cent in the control facilities. Ray *et al.* (1997) used a paired $t$-test at the cluster level to conclude that the observed effect of intervention in these data is statistically significant ($p = 0.03$). While the mean rate of injurious falls is also lower for intervention facilities (13.7 falls per 100 person-years) than for control facilities (19.9 falls per 100 person-years), this difference is not statistically significant, again based on a paired $t$-test performed at the cluster level ($p = 0.22$). Similar conclusions were also reached using exact permutation tests, consistent with the results of simulation studies reported by Brookmeyer and Chen (1998). These authors also proposed a two-stage regression approach which may be used to adjust for imbalance on baseline covariates not accounted for by random assignment.

**Table 8.3** Summary data from a matched-pair trial of a consultation service to reduce falls among residents (Ray *et al.* 1997)

| | Intervention group | | | | | |
|---|---|---|---|---|---|---|
| | Experimental | | | Control | | |
| Nursing home pair | Number of study residents | Recurrent faller (%) | Injurious falls (per 100 person-years) | Number of study residents | Recurrent faller (%) | Injurious falls (per 100 person-years) |
| 1 | 29 | 53.4 | 19.0 | 27 | 63.0 | 16.6 |
| 2 | 27 | 34.4 | 8.1 | 32 | 45.7 | 7.4 |
| 3 | 40 | 54.2 | 8.4 | 33 | 57.7 | 30.5 |
| 4 | 28 | 29.1 | 9.0 | 55 | 46.4 | 14.9 |
| 5 | 18 | 49.2 | 7.0 | 24 | 60.9 | 28.5 |
| 6 | 43 | 57.1 | 27.8 | 50 | 51.4 | 18.1 |
| 7 | 36 | 28.7 | 16.8 | 40 | 53.9 | 23.1 |
| Mean | | 43.7 | 13.7 | | 54.1 | 19.9 |

## 8.2 Categorical data

In this section, we consider methods for the analysis of ordinal and nominal outcome data. Outcome variables which can be ordered but which are not associated with any specific numerical values are said to be measured on an ordinal scale. Data are said to be measured on a nominal scale when observations can be classified into categories but when the categories are not ordered. We focus attention here on outcomes which can be classified into any one of three or more categories, since binary outcome data (a special case of both ordinal and nominal outcome data) were considered in Chapter 6.

An example of ordinal outcome data is provided by Howard-Pitney *et al.* (1997) in their trial of a dietary fat intervention for low-literacy adults. Study subjects were drawn from 24 vocational training and general education classes. Classes were pair-matched on the basis of class size and type, with one class in each of the 12 pairs randomly assigned to receive a programme which focused specifically on the lowering of dietary fat intake, while the control class received a more general nutrition programme. Among the outcomes of interest were several items concerned with nutritional attitudes, each recorded on a five-point scale (1 = strongly agree, 5 = strongly disagree). Analyses of these outcomes were conducted at the cluster level using a paired *t*-test to compare mean scores across intervention groups.

Since the decision to assign values from 1 through 5 is totally arbitrary, differences in the average scores across intervention groups cannot be directly interpreted. Difficulties such as these have sometimes prompted investigators to use non-parametric hypothesis tests and to omit the construction of confidence intervals. However, even cluster-level analyses based on non-parametric tests may be problematic in this context. Suppose, for example, that the investigators above used a non-parametric procedure to compare nutritional attitude scores by computing the average value of cluster-specific summary measures such as the cluster mean or median. It is easily seen that the arbitrary assignment of individual-level scores complicates the ordering of clusters based on summary measures. These and other difficulties in the ordering of clusters using ordinal data have been addressed by Fay and Gennings (1996), who propose a non-parametric procedure which yields results independent of the individual-level scores.

For individually randomized trials, standard methods for the analysis of categorical data (Rosner 1995, Section 10.8) can be used to test for the effect of intervention when outcomes are nominal or ordinal, such as the Pearson chi-square test. In Chapter 6 we presented a simple adjustment which can be applied to this test to account for the effects of clustering when outcomes are binary. Similar adjustments have also been developed for nominal outcome data, as discussed by Rao and Thomas (1988). However, these relatively more complex procedures may require the use of specialized software, e.g. SUDAAN (Shah *et al.* 1996, Ch. 6).

Extensions of logistic regression models for nominal and ordinal outcomes are now widely available. Ananth and Kleinbaum (1997) provide a useful introduction to these procedures, which unfortunately are only applicable when subjects' responses are independent. However, methods to adjust these procedures for the effects of clustering have also been developed. For example, the package SUDAAN (Shah *et al.* 1996, Ch. 15) may be used to fit both ordinal and polytomous logistic regression models while adjusting for the effects of clustering using a version of the GEE robust variance estimator.

Hedeker and Gibbons (1996) describe an alternative approach that can be used to adjust ordinal logistic regression models for the effect of clustering. Their methods are illustrated in the context of a school-based cluster randomization trial examining the effect of a smoking prevention and cessation programme aimed at adolescents (Flay *et al.* 1995). Between-cluster variability is accounted for by the inclusion of a random variable on the logit scale, yielding a model analogous to the mixed-effects logistic regression model described in Section 6.2. One limitation of this approach is that the resulting estimates of intervention effect may be difficult to interpret (Ten Have *et al.* 1996).

Additional research is needed to evaluate the performance of these methods as applied to cluster randomization trials. However, existing research on methods for analysing correlated binary data suggest that they require a relatively large number of clusters in each intervention group.

# 9

# Reporting of cluster randomization trials

Reporting standards for randomized clinical trials have now been widely disseminated (e.g. Begg *et al.* 1996). Many of the principles that apply to trials randomizing individuals also apply to trials randomizing intact clusters. These include a carefully posed justification for the trial, a clear statement of the study objectives and a detailed description of the planned intervention. Other requirements include precise definitions of the primary and secondary endpoints, a description of the method of randomization and an accurate accounting of all subjects randomized to the trial. Unambiguous inclusion–exclusion criteria must also be formulated, although perhaps separately for cluster-level and individual-level characteristics. There are, however, some unique aspects of cluster randomization trials that require special attention at the reporting stage. These include the need to justify the decision to randomize clusters rather than individuals, and an explanation of how the effects of clustering were accounted for in the determination of sample size and the construction of inferences concerning the effect of intervention. In this chapter we discuss these and other relevant issues from the point of view of writing a final trial report. A corresponding summary of guidelines is given in Table 9.1. Section 9.1 discusses the issues that arise in the reporting of study design, while Section 9.2 deals with the reporting of study results.

## 9.1 Reporting of study design

The decreased statistical efficiency of cluster randomization relative to individual randomization can be substantial, depending on the sizes of the clusters randomized and the degree of within-cluster resemblance. Thus, unless there is obviously no alternative, the reasons for randomizing clusters rather than individuals should be clearly stated. This information, accompanied by a clear description of the units randomized, can help a reader to decide if the loss of precision due to cluster randomization is in fact justified.

Having decided to randomize clusters, investigators may still have considerable latitude in their choice of unit. As first noted in Section 3.2, this decision is not always straightforward. Given the varied levels of statistical efficiency associated with different cluster sizes, it would seem important to select the unit of randomization

**Table 9.1** Guidelines for statistical reporting of cluster randomization trials

*Reporting of study design*
1. Justify the use of cluster randomization.
2. Provide a clear definition of the unit of randomization.
3. Indicate whether inferences are primarily directed at the cluster level or at the level of the individual subject.
4. Describe the process of consent used for (i) randomizing clusters, and (ii) collecting data from study participants.
5. Describe the experimental design (e.g. completely randomized, stratified, matched-pair) and the method of randomization.
6. Explain how the chosen sample size or statistical power calculations accounts for between-cluster variation.

*Reporting of study results*
1. Provide the number of clusters randomized, the average cluster size and the number of subjects selected for study from each cluster.
2. Provide the values of the intracluster correlation coefficient as calculated for the primary outcome variables.
3. Compare the baseline characteristics of the intervention groups at both the individual and the cluster level.
4. Explain how the reported statistical analyses account for between-cluster variation.
5. Describe how prognostically important baseline risk factors were adjusted for.
6. Report on loss to follow-up of both individuals within clusters and entire clusters.

on a carefully considered basis. However, it is apparent from published reports that this may not always have been the case. For example, the review of cluster randomization studies reported by Donner *et al.* (1990) found that only one-quarter of the trials considered provided reasons for their choice of randomization unit. An unambiguous definition of the unit of randomization is also required. Thus a statement that 'neighbourhoods' were randomized is clearly incomplete without a detailed description of this term in the context of the planned trial.

An accurate and detailed description of the study aims is important in any comparative trial. However, this issue is particularly complicated in trials randomizing clusters, not only because the interventions are often inherently complex, but also because the natural target of inference could be at either the individual or cluster level (see Section 1.5). Since the choice of inferential unit may influence both the design and analysis of the study, as well as how its results should be interpreted, this issue should be clarified very early in the trial report.

In some cases, the detailed components of a complex intervention may be systematically planned using the cooperation of several relevant stakeholders. For example, Fisher (1995), in an editorial concerning community intervention trials, discussed how investigators might collaborate with selected members of the community to help develop and refine the final intervention. Collaboration of this type could then result in an intervention which, to various degrees, is 'tailored' to fit the population of interest, ideally in a manner driven by an overall theoretic framework (Sorensen *et al.* 1998). Such collaboration was an integral part of the British Family Heart Study (Marteau *et al.* 1996), where a change in lifestyle was negotiated individually for each intervention subject, depending upon the subject's assessed quintile of risk for coronary disease as compared with others of the same age and sex. However, detailed tailoring of interventions is also seen in worksite trials. For example, the intervention in the Take-Heart programme (Glasgow *et al.* 1995b) was designed to maximize the fit between the programme content and existing worksite norms, with detailed activities developed and planned in accordance with a carefully specified model.

It is clear that in trials as complex as those described above, careful description is needed to adequately convey the content of the intervention as it is actually delivered, whether administered directly to individual subjects or implemented at the cluster level. Otherwise, it may be impossible to accurately generalize the results to other populations. If the description is incomplete or vague, there is even a risk that it may be difficult for readers to decide what the intervention actually comprised. Some discussion should also be provided as to any potential co-intervention (e.g. a new medical initiative undertaken in a community) or source of contamination that may have skewed the intended delivery of the intervention.

For reasons discussed in Chapter 4, the consensus that exists in most clinical trial settings regarding the role of informed consent has not tended to apply in trials randomizing intact clusters. For instance, in many community intervention trials this issue has been ignored entirely, while in others it has sometimes been regarded as ethically acceptable if decisions involving random assignment and implementation of the intervention are made by community leaders. This is in contrast to trials involving smaller clusters, such as families or households, where informed consent has frequently been obtained from each eligible subject. By reporting the methods used (if any) to obtain informed consent in their own trials, it may gradually become possible for the research community to develop reasonably uniform standards regarding this important issue.

The clusters that participate in a trial, simply owing to their consent to be randomized, may not be representative of the target population of clusters. Some indication of this lack of representativeness may be obtained by listing the number of clusters that met the eligibility criteria for the trial, but which declined to participate, along with a description of their characteristics.

The CONSORT statement (Begg *et al.* 1996) recommends reporting the method used to generate the intervention assignment. In cluster randomization trials, this will often consist of a computer program for generating random numbers used to allocate clusters to either an experimental or a control group. An example of such a detailed description is given in the nursing trial reported by Gilliss *et al.* (1993), who used a random permuted-blocks scheme (Pocock 1983, Section 5.2) to control for possible changes in the hospital patient population and care-giver practice over time. The description of the randomization scheme should also be given in the context of the experimental design adopted (e.g. completely randomized, matched-pair, stratified). In the trial referred to above (Gilliss *et al.* 1993), the permuted-blocks randomization scheme was implemented separately within each of two hospital strata, with the intervention assignment not known to the investigators enrolling the patients. The investigators also noted that the random assignment of a cluster 'was not disclosed until a patient in the cluster had reached a point in the trial where the experimental intervention differed from the control'. Information such as this is very helpful in allowing a reader to evaluate the impact of blinding restrictions on the reported conclusions.

Administrative realities sometimes require that an intervention be introduced gradually over a period of time to newly accrued units. This was the case, for example, in the HIV prevention trial reported by Hayes *et al.* (1995) and Grosskurth *et al.*

(1995), which required a period of 2 months to introduce each pair of matched communities into the trial, and with a total of 12 months required to enter all six pairs. A follow-up survey was conducted in each pair of communities 2 years after an initial baseline survey was conducted.

This type of detailed information comprises what Begg *et al.* (1996) refer to as the 'trial profile'. If it also provides a description of the timing of the randomization for each cluster, with similar information given for the introduction of the intervention and the measurements, it will allow the reader to make a more careful judgement as to both the internal and external validity of the reported conclusions.

It was mentioned in Section 1.1 that cluster randomization is sometimes adopted as a means of avoiding experimental contamination. However, the risk of contamination, although perhaps reduced as compared with trials randomizing individuals, may still be present. In community trials, for example, individuals living in a control community may travel to an experimental community, either specifically to take advantage of what may be perceived as improved services, or simply as a result of normal migratory patterns. In trials randomizing medical practices or clinics, there might also be a risk that colleagues share information or that staff who administer the intervention come into contact with patients allocated to the other arm of the trial. Where relevant, it is therefore useful to report what steps were taken to reduce the possibility of such contamination. These steps could include measures taken to disguise subjects' awareness of the specific intervention administered, the adoption of a randomization scheme that assures a reasonable degree of physical separation between clusters in different arms of the trial, or the allocation of personnel in such a way as to minimize the possibility that subjects receive treatment from ineligible staff. It is difficult to monitor the exact extent to which such measures will be successful, but some progress can often be made through careful follow-up and cooperation between participating centres. For example, in the HIV prevention trial reported by Hayes *et al.* (1995) and Grosskurth *et al.* (1995), data on place of residence were collected at participating health facilities as a method of tracking individuals who might have migrated from one arm of the trial to the other.

A continuing difficulty with reports of randomized trials is that justification for the sample size is all too often omitted (Moher *et al.* 1994). These omissions are particularly problematic for trials in which the effect of intervention is substantively but not statistically significant. It is then difficult to determine if the trial was negative because it was underpowered, or, as is often assumed, because the intervention was ineffective. The risk of designing an underpowered trial is even greater when adopting cluster randomization, since administrative and financial concerns often limit the number of clusters which can be randomized. As noted in Chapter 5, the trial may also be underpowered because the presence of intracluster correlation was not considered in the determination of sample size. Investigators should therefore clearly describe how the sample size for their trial was determined, with particular attention given to how clustering effects were adjusted for. This description should be in the context of the experimental design selected (e.g. completely randomized, matched-pair, stratified) and should indicate whether the sample size calculations were based on a one- or two-sided statistical test.

If only a subsample of subjects are selected for study within each cluster, the size of this subsample should also be reported, along with the sampling method used. For stratified designs, investigators should report both the number of subjects and the number of clusters in each combination of intervention group and stratum.

It should be emphasized that reporting the sample size for a trial solely in terms of the number of subjects is in a sense misleading, since it might be taken to imply that the study has a greater degree of information than is actually the case. This is because the effective sample size for a given trial is really the stated number of subjects divided by the design effect (see Section 5.2.1 for a worked example). The concept of effective sample size may be particularly important if it is of interest to compare the amount of information supplied by a study randomizing villages, for example, with that supplied by a study randomizing individuals. In this case, it is appropriate to compare the effective sample size for the two studies as well as the actual number of subjects.

It should be further specified what provisions, if any, were made in the sample size calculations to account for potential loss to follow-up. Since the factors leading to the loss to follow-up of individual members of a cluster may be very different from those leading to the loss of an entire cluster, both sets of factors must be considered here.

While most trials have attempted to allocate an equal number of clusters to each intervention group, some investigators have deliberately chosen to adopt an unbalanced allocation scheme. For example, the CATCH, first described in Chapter 1 (Zucker *et al.* 1995) systematically allocated more schools to the experimental group than to the control group. One reason for adopting such a scheme might be to help secure the cooperation of school officials, who are then assured a greater than 50:50 chance of receiving the experimental intervention. However, given the potential lack of efficiency of this design relative to a design randomizing the same number of clusters to each group, the underlying rationale for this decision should be clearly stated.

## 9.2 Reporting of study results

The relatively small effective sample size that characterizes many cluster randomization trials implies that the probability of imbalance between intervention groups on prognostically important baseline variables may be substantial. Reports of cluster randomization trials should therefore include a table showing the baseline distribution of important characteristics by intervention group. The information in this table provides a check on the effectiveness of the randomization as well as an indication as to which baseline characteristics should be adjusted for. Since the generalizability of the trial results may be determined both by the characteristics of individual participants (e.g. age, sex) and by the characteristics of clusters (e.g. type of worksite), it is advisable to report the table in two sections, one showing the comparability of individual-level characteristics and the other showing the comparability of cluster-level characteristics. This baseline table should include the number of clusters randomized and the average cluster size (and possibly the range of cluster sizes) in each group, since the overall precision of the study depends on both these quantities.

The use of significance tests alone for comparing baseline characteristics between intervention groups is a common error in all randomized trials (e.g. Begg 1990, Senn 1994). This error arises because, under a properly executed randomization scheme, any observed baseline difference can only be a result of chance, thus negating the main purpose of performing a significance test. The problem is compounded in cluster randomization trials that compare individual-level characteristics without taking into account the clustering, as the resulting $p$-values will be spuriously low. It is the magnitude of the baseline differences and the predictive relationship of the baseline variable with the trial outcome measure which should govern the decision as to whether adjustment is required. Nonetheless, the reporting of (properly computed) $p$-values as a descriptive measure can still serve a useful purpose in signalling what baseline characteristics are not well balanced. In this case the fairly common practice of using symbols such as 'NS' for 'not significant' is of limited helpfulness and should be replaced by the actual $p$-values, properly adjusted for clustering.

If baseline standard deviations are presented for descriptive purposes, then it should be made clear as to whether these are crude between-subject standard deviations computed across all clusters in an intervention group, or whether (as would be theoretically preferable) they take into account both between- and within-cluster components of variation. Reporting the range of baseline variables rather than standard deviations is a simple way of avoiding this potential problem of interpretation, with, admittedly, some loss of information.

It was noted in Chapter 5 that investigators are frequently hampered in planning the size of cluster randomization trials by a lack of prior information concerning the likely value of the intracluster correlation coefficient $\rho$. A statistically justified sample size assessment is not possible without an advance estimate of this parameter. Thus it would be beneficial to the research community if empirical estimates of $\rho$ were routinely published (with an indication of whether or not the reported values have been adjusted for the effect of baseline covariates). This would not only help researchers who are designing new trials in a similar subject matter area, but would also allow a greater understanding of how the magnitude of this parameter varies according to different units of randomization in different subject populations. For trials involving more than one level of nesting, the value of the intracluster correlation at each level should be reported. A complete report would also provide the values of the between- and within-components of variance separately for each intracluster correlation.

Investigators have sometimes reported design effects, which are a function of both average cluster size and the level of intracluster correlation, rather than the value of the intracluster correlation itself. This is clearly not as informative as listing the two components of the design effect separately, and may thus hamper the planning of future trials.

For stratified designs, some indication of the benefit of stratification and/or matching could be reported in order to help in the planning of future trials. This could include, for example, the reporting of simple Pearson correlation coefficients between the success rates of experimental and control group patients assigned to the same match or stratum. Table 3.2 (p. 37) displays these correlations for a selected number of matched-pair trials.

Confidence intervals are useful in any study for providing a measure of the uncertainty with which intervention effects are estimated. However, they may be particularly valuable in reporting the results of cluster randomization trials. As indicated in the reviews cited in Section 1.2, such trials are frequently underpowered and thus likely to be statistically non-significant even in the presence of important intervention effects. It is well-known (e.g. Gardner and Altman 1986) that the interpretation of non-significant results from comparative trials is enhanced by their presentation in terms of confidence limits. However, the construction of such limits must take into account the effect of clustering, since the resulting intervals may otherwise be spuriously narrow.

As indicated in Chapters 6–8, a large variety of methods, based on very different sets of assumptions, have been used to analyse data arising from cluster randomization trials. For example, possible choices for the analysis of dichotomous outcomes include adjusted chi-square statistics, the method of generalized estimating equations (GEE) and logistic-normal regression models. These methods are not as familiar as the standard procedures commonly used to analyse clinical trial data. This is partly because methodology for analysing cluster randomization trials is in a state of rapid development, with virtually no standardization and a proliferation of associated software. Therefore, it is incumbent on authors to provide a clear statement of the statistical methods used, accompanied, where it is not obvious, by an explanation of how the analysis adjusts for the effect of clustering. The software used to implement these analyses should also be reported.

Whichever method of analysis is selected, it should be made clear that the intent-to-treat approach has been used for the primary analysis, i.e. that this analysis includes all cluster members followed up in each randomized group, regardless of the intervention actually received. This implies, for example, that subjects who leave their cluster will nonetheless be followed and counted in the analysis, as will all other subjects who provide data. Secondary analyses in which certain clusters or cluster members are not counted (sometimes called efficacy analyses) can also be informative, but are generally less credible, since they are not protected by the randomization.

Unfortunately, analyses done by intent-to-treat may be difficult to interpret when practical considerations directly affect the ability of investigators to adhere to the randomization scheme. This is not an uncommon problem. For example, as discussed in Section 5.5, the review of primary prevention trials by Simpson *et al.* (1995) found that in some studies, clusters were reassigned to their intervention after randomization, while in other studies clusters simply did not receive the intended intervention. When this serious form of non-adherence occurs, the credibility of the trial conclusions is clearly enhanced if they are supported by the results of several different analyses that make different assumptions.

In general, the effect of low compliance among subjects assigned to the experimental group will tend to dilute estimated treatment effects. As noted by Paci and Alexander (1997), however, estimating the actual impact of non-compliance on the trial results may be difficult. Nonetheless, the quantitative assessment of subject and staff compliance to all relevant aspects of the trial protocol, where feasible, may be crucial to interpreting these results.

Special difficulties of interpretation arise in the analysis of trials designed to show 'equivalence'. In this case, the intent-to-treat analysis may be no longer conservative, and efficacy analyses should therefore play a more prominent role (e.g. see Jones *et al.* 1996). These analyses could systematically exclude, for example, clusters and/or subjects that showed a high degree of non-compliance to their assigned intervention. If the results of these analyses continue to support the claim of equivalence, the overall credibility of this claim will be enhanced.

In spite of intense efforts at avoiding losses to follow-up, it is inevitable in large cohort trials that data on some subjects will be missing. As in any randomized trial, the authors should report the discrepancy between the number of subjects entering the trial and the number analysed in each intervention group. Moreover, if entire clusters have been lost to follow-up, this should be reported separately from losses to follow-up of individuals within clusters. As suggested by the CONSORT statement, this information can be presented as part of a flow chart marking the progress of subjects through a randomized trial. However, the CONSORT illustration of a flow chart (e.g. Begg *et al.* 1996) is strictly applicable only to individually randomized trials. An interesting example of a flow chart which reports both the progress of clusters and that of subjects within clusters is provided by Auleley *et al.* (1997, Fig. 1), as based on their hospital randomized trial which examined the effect of practice guidelines on the treatment of patients with ankle injuries.

Simply reporting the overall loss to follow-up rates in each group provides no information as to whether the losses predominantly come from one or two clusters or are more or less evenly distributed across the clusters in a group. This information is particularly valuable in studies involving only a few large aggregate units, where the losses may be largely concentrated in those units having special characteristics.

Given the uncertainty of interpretation frequently associated with trials having appreciable levels of attrition, the reasons for the loss to follow-up should be discussed in the context of its potential impact on the validity of the stated trial conclusions. As in clinical trials randomizing individuals, this impact is likely to be minimal provided the reasons for loss to follow-up are unrelated to the assigned intervention. Loss to follow-up rates that are markedly different in the two groups would present strong evidence against this assumption.

Similar care should be taken when describing participation rates in trials conducted using cross-sectional surveys. Trial conclusions will be particularly suspect if participation rates vary across intervention groups.

The approach taken to handle missing data can be critical to properly interpreting the trial results, particularly if the loss to follow-up rate is large, and therefore should be described in detail. Various strategies may be considered, including imputation techniques which assign numerical estimates to the missing values. These techniques could include mean substitution, 'last value forward', or the use of regression methods, none of which correctly accounts for the effect of imputation on the resulting estimates of variance. However, more sophisticated methods have also been described in which the uncertainty of imputed values is accounted for by using multiple estimates for each missing observation (e.g. Heitjan 1997).

Since all such strategies are subject to the potential criticism that the missing data are 'made up', performing several such analyses is advisable, including one in which those subjects with missing data are simply removed. As an example, the CATCH (Zucker *et al.* 1995) formulated in advance a large number of 'sensitivity' analyses, where each analysis allowed different assumptions about how the missing data might affect the study conclusions. If the trial conclusions remain stable across different sets of assumptions, their overall credibility is clearly strengthened. In this case a supplementary table which describes the differences in baseline characteristics between those subjects with and without endpoint data would be useful.

It is natural in the analysis of data arising from any major trial to explore how the effect of intervention varies among different subgroups of subjects. In the case of matched-pair or stratified cluster randomization trials, for example, it may be of interest to identify, albeit in an exploratory manner, those strata in which the intervention appears to be most beneficial. Subgroup analyses defined by categorized values of individual-level covariates, or a mixture of individual-level and cluster-level covariates, may also be of interest. For example, Green (1997) reports how the effect of the implemented smoking cessation intervention in the COMMIT trial varied by categorized levels of age, sex and educational achievement.

The appropriate strategy for conducting subgroup analyses can be complex, as indicated by the extensive literature on this subject (e.g. Simon 1982, Fleming 1995). Much of this literature focuses on the task of minimizing the risk of finding spurious intervention effects by chance alone, i.e. minimizing the overall type I error rate. Since these guidelines apply with equal force to cluster randomization trials, investigators should be encouraged in their reporting to indicate how the resulting interpretational problems were dealt with. This could include a statement describing how the subgroups of interest were selected, ideally on the basis of previous trial findings or other considerations that allowed their pre-specification in the protocol.

Statistical analyses used to identify subgroup effects should employ tests of interaction or other techniques for controlling overall type I error, such as adopting a more stringent level of statistical significance. The following remark by Pocock (1983, Section 14.1) should also be kept in mind: 'Separate significance tests for different subgroups do not provide direct evidence of whether a prognostic factor affects the treatment difference.' The usefulness of this remark is made clear by appreciating the role of the subgroup sample size involved in the separate significance tests. An intervention effect of modest magnitude may be statistically significant in a given subgroup simply as a result of a large number of clusters or subjects, while an effect of exactly the same magnitude in a different subgroup may be non-significant owing to a smaller sample size. This problem does not arise if a test of interaction is performed, since then the magnitudes of the intervention effect in the different subgroups are directly compared.

As indicated above, published guidelines regarding the interpretation of subgroup analyses focus for the most part on controlling the overall type I error rate. However, interpretational problems may also arise concerning the size of type II errors. This is because very few trials are designed to have sufficient power to detect substantively important intervention effects in other than the full sample of subjects. Thus the lack of statistical significance in a given subgroup must always be regarded with caution, since this finding cannot be used in itself to conclude that the intervention is ineffective. Such caution is particularly warranted in cluster randomization trials, since the effective sample size in a given subgroup may be substantially less than the observed sample size. Confidence intervals constructed about the intervention effect observed in a given subgroup have a particularly helpful role to play here.

The typically large investment involved in most cluster randomization trials, combined with their complexity, often leads to a temptation to report the results of analyses conducted on a very large number of endpoints. Although this practice can be quite informative given the multifaceted nature of a subject's response to intervention, it also gives rise to yet further problems of multiplicity. These problems raise a number of interpretational issues that have been extensively discussed in the clinical trials literature (e.g. Tang *et al.* 1993). One of the chief challenges, as in the case of multiple subgroup analyses, is to control the increased likelihood of 'false positives'. Perhaps the most useful overall advice in this regard is provided by Pocock (1983, Section 14.3), who emphasizes the importance of specifying in advance some priority for the various endpoints. Thus two or three relatively independent endpoints, each being of fundamental interest and serving as the basis of the trial design, could be specified as primary, with the remaining endpoints classified as secondary. The term 'relatively independent' in this context implies that these endpoints address different questions, with highly correlated outcomes either reduced in number or combined into a single index. It could then be made clear in the trial report that while analyses conducted on the primary endpoints may be regarded as 'confirmatory', the remaining analyses should be regarded as exploratory or suggestive only. This strategy was adopted in the antenatal care trial described in Chapter 5 (Villar *et al.* 1998), where fetal low birthweight and a maternal morbidity index were selected as the primary response variables, with several other variables explicitly classified as secondary. The trial was sufficiently powered to detect intervention group differences only with respect to the primary outcome variables.

Similar problems arise when reporting the results of significance tests performed over a series of subject follow-ups, corresponding, for example, to annual assessments over a period spanning several years. To help control the overall type I error rate arising in this context, some authors have adopted a more stringent significance level for each test reported. For example, Chou *et al.* (1998) used a significance level of $\alpha = 0.004$ in reporting the results of analyses performed at four separate follow-up occasions in their community-level cohort study. An alternative strategy is to perform significance tests only at the most meaningful time point, such as at the end of the last follow-up period, regarding the intermediate analyses as of descriptive interest only.

In stating the trial conclusions, it is helpful to discuss the external validity or generalizability of the results. The extent to which the results are generalizable depends to some extent on the degree of control that the subject has over his or her compliance with the intervention. Where care-givers are involved, the outcome of the intervention may also depend to a certain extent on the person providing the care. As discussed by Black (1996), the outcome of a pharmaceutical intervention is to a large extent unaffected by the characteristics of the prescribing doctor. Pharmaceutical trials also tend to have established standardized procedures for monitoring compliance. This is usually not the case for non-therapeutic trials evaluating interventions such as mass education, different forms of patient management, changes in the workplace, economic programmes or shifts in policy. The outcome measures from these trials may in fact be highly dependent on the characteristics of the provider, setting and subjects. Yet these are precisely the types of interventions that tend to be the focus of cluster randomization trials, and therefore it is important to discuss the extent to which their results may be safely generalized. For example, investigators may be concerned that care-givers who agree to participate in a trial are fairly unrepresentative, since their degree of interest in the topic and level of enthusiasm may be unusually high.

Investigators are also often interested in comparing their results with those of previously conducted cluster randomized trials. A complicating factor in making such comparisons is that all too often the earlier investigators failed to account for the impact of clustering. One simple, but admittedly approximate, strategy is to multiply variance estimators of the observed intervention effect by the inflation factor $IF = 1 + (\overline{m} - 1)\rho$, where the mean cluster size, $\overline{m}$, is obtained from the earlier trial and the intracluster correlation coefficient $\rho$ is estimated from current data. Adjusted variance estimates can then be used to correct confidence intervals or test statistics for the impact of clustering. More generally it should be noted that if an unadjusted test statistic fails to reach statistical significance, the appropriate adjustment for clustering will only make it less significant.

Examples of how this strategy has been used in the context of meta-analysis are given by Fawzi *et al.* (1993) and by Rooney and Murray (1996).

# References

Aalen, O.O., Bjertness, E. and Sonju, T. 1995: Analysis of dependent survival data applied to lifetimes of amalgam fillings. *Statistics in Medicine* **14**, 1819–1829.

Abdeljaber, M.H., Monto, A.S., Tilden, R.L., Schork, M.A. and Tarwotjo, I. 1991: The impact of vitamin A supplementation on morbidity: a randomized community intervention trial. *American Journal of Public Health* **81**, 1654–1656.

Ahn, C. and Lee, J. 1997: A computer program for the analysis of over-dispersed counts and proportions. *Computer Methods and Programs in Biomedicine* **52**, 195–202.

Aickin, M. and Ritenbaugh, C. 1991: A criterion for the adequacy of a simple design when a complex model will be used for analysis. *Controlled Clinical Trials* **12**, 560–565.

Alexander, F.E. and Boyle, P. (eds) 1996: Methods for investigating localized clustering of disease. Lyon, France: International Agency for Research on Cancer.

Alexander, F, Roberts, M.M., Lutz, W. and Hepburn, W. 1989: Randomization by cluster and the problem of social class bias. *Journal of Epidemiology and Community Health* **43**, 29–36.

Alexander, S., Belizán, J., Althabe, F. *et al.* 1997: Evaluation of a strategy to control the epidemic of cesarian sections in Latin America (unpubl.).

Altman, D.G. and Bland, J.M. 1991: Improving doctor's understanding of statistics. *Journal of the Royal Statistical Society, Series A* **154**, 223–267.

Altman, D.G. and Goodman, S.N. 1994: Transfer of technology from statistical journals to the biomedical literature. Past trends and future predictions. *Journal of the American Medical Association* **272**, 129–132.

Altman, D.G., Whitehead, J., Parmar, M.K., Stenning, S.P., Fayers, P.M. and Machin, D. 1995: Randomised consent designs in cancer clinical trials. *European Journal of Cancer* **31A** (12), 1934–1944.

Amberson, J.B. Jr, McMahon, B.T. and Pinner, M. 1931: A clinical trial of sanocrysin in pulmonary tuberculosis. *American Review of Tuberculosis* **24**, 401–435.

Ananth, C.V. and Kleinbaum, D.G. 1997: Regression models for ordinal responses: a review of methods and applications. *International Journal of Epidemiology* **26**, 1323–1333.

Andersen, B. 1990: *Methodological errors in medical research: an incomplete catalogue*. Oxford: Blackwell Scientific Publications.

Apostolides, A. and Henderson, M. 1977: Evaluation of cancer screening programs: parallels with clinical trials. *Cancer* **39**, 1779–1785.

Armitage, P. 1972: History of randomised controlled trials. *Lancet* **1**, 1388.

Armitage, P. 1982: The role of randomization in clinical trials. *Statistics in Medicine* **1**, 345–352.

Armitage, P. and Berry, G. 1994: *Statistical methods in medical research*, 3rd edn. Oxford: Blackwell Scientific Publications.

Ashby, M., Neuhaus, J.M., Hauck, W.W *et al.* 1992: An annotated bibliography of methods for analyzing correlated categorical data. *Statistics in Medicine* **11**, 67–99.

Auleley, G.R., Ravaud, P., Giraudeau, B. *et al.* 1997: Implementation of the Ottawa ankle rules in France. A multicenter randomized controlled trial. *Journal of the American Medical Association* **277,** 1935–1939.

Avorn, J. 1992: Letter to the editor. *New England Journal of Medicine* **327**, 1393.

Avorn, J., Soumeri, S.B., Everitt, D.E. *et al.* 1992: A randomized trial of a program to reduce the use of psychoactive drugs in nursing homes. *New England Journal of Medicine* **327**, 168–173.

Baranowski, T., Lin, L.S., Wetter, D.W., Bresnicow, K. and Hearn, M.D. 1997: Theory as mediating variables: why aren't community interventions working as desired? *Annals of Epidemiology* Supplement 7, S89–S95.

Barcikowski, R.S. 1981: Statistical power with group mean as the unit of analysis. *Journal of Educational Statistics* **6**, 267–285.

Bass, M.J., McWhinney, I.R. and Donner A. 1986: Do family physicians need medical assistants to detect and manage hypertension? *Canadian Medical Association Journal* **134**, 1247–1255.

Begg, C.B. 1990: Significance tests of covariate imbalance in clinical trials. *Controlled Clinical Trials* **11**, 223–225.

Begg, C., Cho, M., Eastwood, S. *et al.* 1996: Improving the quality of reporting of randomized controlled trials, The CONSORT statement. *Journal of the American Medical Association* **276**, 637–639.

Bennett, C.A. and Lumsdaine, A.A. 1975: *Evaluation and experiment. Some critical issues in assessing social programs.* New York: Academic Press.

Berelson, B. and Freedman, R. 1964: A study in fertility control. *Scientific American* **210**, 29–37.

Bergman, A.B. and Stamm, S.J. 1967: The morbidity of cardiac nondisease in school children. *New England Journal of Medicine* **276**, 1008–1013.

Berkow, R. 1992: *The Merck manual of diagnosis and therapy*, 16th edn. Rahway, NJ: Merck.

Black, N. 1996: Why we need observational studies to evaluate the effectiveness of health care. *British Medical Journal* **312**, 1215–1218.

Blair, R.C. and Higgins, J.J. 1986: Comment on statistical power with group mean as the unit of analysis. *Journal of Educational Statistics* **11**, 161–169.

Bland, J.M. and Kerry, S.M. 1997: Statistics notes. Trials randomised in clusters. *British Medical Journal* **315**, 600.

Bland, J.M. and Kerry, S.M. 1998: Statistics notes. Weighted comparison of means. *British Medical Journal* **316**, 129.

Bloom, B.S. 1986: Controlled studies in measuring the efficacy of medical care: a historical perspective. *International Journal of Technology Assessment in Health Care* **2**, 299–310.

Blum, D. and Feachem, R.G. 1983: Measuring the impact of water supply and sanitation investments on diarrhoeal diseases: problems of methodology. *International Journal of Epidemiology* **12**, 357–365.

Boos, D.D. 1992: On generalized score tests. *American Statistician* **46**, 327–333.

Boruch, R.F., McSweeny, A.J. and Soderstrom, E.J. 1978: Randomized field experiments for program planning, development, and evaluation. *Evaluation Quarterly* **2**, 655–695.

Breslow, N. 1976: Regression analysis of the log odds ratio: a method for retrospective studies. *Biometrics* **32**, 409–416.

Breslow, N.E. 1984: Extra-Poisson variation in log-linear models. *Applied Statistics* **33**, 38–44.

Breslow, N.E. and Day, N.E. 1987: *Statistical methods in cancer research, Volume II – the design and analysis of cohort studies.* Lyons: International Agency for Research on Cancer.

Brier, S.S. 1980: Analysis of contingency tables under cluster sampling. *Biometrika* **67**, 591–596.

Brook, R.H, Ware, J.E. Jr, Rogers, W.H. *et al.* 1983: Does free care improve adults' health? Results from a randomized controlled trial. *New England Journal of Medicine* **309**, 1426–1434.

Brookmeyer, R. and Chen, Y-Q. 1998: Person-time analysis of paired community intervention trials when the number of communities is small. *Statistics in Medicine* **17**, 2121–2132.

Brown, R.L., Baumann, L.J., Helberg, C.P., Han, Y., Fontana, S.A. and Love, R.R. 1996: The simultaneous analysis of patient, physician and group practice influences on annual mammography performance. *Social Science and Medicine* **43**, 315–324.

Brownson, R.C., Newschaffer, C.J. and Ali-Abarghoui, F. 1997: Policy research for disease prevention: challenges and practical recommendations. *American Journal of Public Health* **87**, 735–739.

Bryk, A.S. and Raudenbush, S.W. 1992: *Hierarchical linear models: application and data analysis methods*. Newbury Park: Sage Publications.

Buck, C. and Donner, A. 1982: The design of controlled experiments in the evaluation of non-therapeutic interventions. *Journal of Chronic Diseases* **35**, 531–538.

Buiatti E. 1996: Evaluation of human trial design, In Stewart, B.W., McGregor, D. and Kleihues, P. (eds), *Principles of chemoprevention*. Scientific Publication No. 139. Lyon: International Agency for Research on Cancer, 261–269.

Bullough, C.H., Msuku, R.S. and Karonde, L. 1989: Early suckling and postpartum haemorrhage: controlled trial in deliveries by traditional birth attendants. *Lancet* **2**, 522–525.

Burstein, L. and Smith, I.D. 1977: Choosing the appropriate unit for investigating school effects. *Australian Journal of Education* **21**, 65–79.

Butler, C. and Bachmann, M. 1996: Design and analysis of studies evaluating smoking cessation interventions where effects vary between practices or practitioners. *Family Practice* **13**, 402–407.

Byar, D. 1988: The design of cancer prevention trials. *Recent Results in Cancer Research* **111**, 3–48.

Cambien, F., Richard, J.L., Jacqueson, A. and Ducimetiere, P. 1981: Analysis of the results of a trial where groups have been randomized, The Paris cardiovascular prevention trial. *Revue Epidémiologique et Santé Publique* **29**, 281–288.

Campbell, D.T. and Stanley, J.C. 1963: *Experimental and quasi-experimental designs for research*. Chicago: Rand McNally College Publishing.

Carleton, R.A., Lasater, T.M., Assaf, A.R., Feldman, H.A. and McKinlay S. 1995: The Pawtucket Heart Health Program: community changes in cardiovascular risk factors and projected disease risk. *American Journal of Public Health* **85**, 777–785.

Chalmers, T.C. and Schroeder, B. 1979: Controls in journal articles. *New England Journal of Medicine* **301**, 1293.

Chen, W., Srinivasan, S.R., Bao, W., Wattigney, W.A. and Berenson, G.S. 1997: Sibling aggregation of low- and high-density lipoprotein cholesterol and apolipoproteins B and A-1 levels in black and white children: the Bogalusa heart study. *Ethnicity and Disease* **7**, 241–249.

Chosidow, O., Chastang, C., Brue, C. *et al.* 1994: Controlled study of malathion and d-phenothrin lotions for *Pediculus humanus* var *capitis* – infested schoolchildren. *Lancet* **344**, 1724–1727.

Chou, C-P., Montgomery, S., Pentz, M.A. *et al.* 1998: Effects of a community-based prevention program on decreasing drug use in high-risk adolescents. *American Journal of Public Health* **88**, 944–948.

Cochran, W.G. 1943: Analysis of variance for percentages based on unequal numbers. *Journal of the American Statistical Association* **38**, 287–301.

Cochran, W.G. 1953: *Sampling techniques*, 2nd edn. New York: John Wiley.

Cochran, W.G. 1977: *Sampling techniques*, 3rd edn. New York: John Wiley.

Cohen, J. 1983: The cost of dichotomization. *Applied Psychological Measurement* **7**, 249–253.

Cohen, J. 1988: *Statistical power analysis for the behavioral sciences*, 2nd edn. Hillsdale, NJ: Academic Press.

COMMIT Research Group. 1995a: Community Intervention Trial for Smoking Cessation (COMMIT): I. Cohort results from a four-year community intervention. *American Journal of Public Health* **85**, 183–192.

COMMIT Research Group.1995b: Community Intervention Trial for Smoking Cessation (COMMIT): II. Changes in adult cigarette smoking prevalence. *American Journal of Public Health* **85**, 193–200.

Comstock, G.W. 1962: Isoniazid prophylaxis in an undeveloped area. *American Review of Respiratory Disease* **86**, 810–822.

Comstock, G.W. 1978: Uncontrolled ruminations on modern controlled trials. *American Journal of Epidemiology* **108**, 81–84.

Conover, W.J. 1980: *Practical nonparametric statistics*, 2nd edn. New York: John Wiley.

Conway, D.J., Hall, A., Anwar, K.S., Rahman, M.L. and Bundy, D.A. 1995: Household aggregation of *Strongyloides stercoralis* infection in Bangladesh. *Transaction of the Royal Society of Tropical Medicine and Hygiene* **89**, 258–261.

Cook, T.D. and Shadish, W.R. 1994: Social experiments: some developments over the past fifteen years. *Annual Review of Psychology* **45**, 545–580.

Coren, S and Hakstian, A.R. 1990: Methodological implications of interaural correlation: count heads not ears. *Perception and Psychophysics* **48**, 291–294

Cornfield, J. 1951: Modern methods in the sampling of human populations. *American Journal of Public Health* **41**, 654–661.

Cornfield, J. 1978: Randomization by group: a formal analysis. *American Journal of Epidemiology* **108**, 100–102.

Cornfield, J. and Mitchell, S. 1969: Selected risk factors in coronary disease. Possible intervention effects. *Archives of Environmental Health* **19**, 382–394.

Council for International Organizations of Medical Sciences (CIOMS) 1991: International guidelines for ethical review of epidemiological studies. In Bankowski, Z., Bryant, J.H. and Last, J.M. (eds), *Ethics and epidemiology: international guidelines. Proceedings of the XXVth CIOMS Conference*. Geneva: CIOMS.

Crain, R.L. 1973: *Southern schools: an evaluation of the effects of the emergency school assistance program and of school desegregation*, vol. I. University of Chicago, Chicago, IL: The National Opinion Research Center.

Cressie, N. 1980: Relaxing assumptions in the one sample *t*-test. *Australian Journal of Statistics* **22**, 143–153.

Cullen, J.W. 1990: Phases in cancer control: intervention research. In Hakama, H., Beral, V., Cullen, J.W. and Parkin, D.M. (eds), *Evaluating effectiveness of primary prevention of cancer*. Scientific Publication No. 103. Lyon: International Agency for Research on Cancer.

D'Arcy Hart, P. 1972: History of randomized control trials. *Lancet* **1**, 965.

Dennis, M. 1997: Commentary: why we didn't ask patients for their consent. *British Medical Journal* **314**, 1077.

Dennis, M., O'Rourke, S., Slattery, J., Staniforth, T. and Warlow, C. 1997: Evaluation of a stroke family care worker: results of a randomised controlled trial. *British Medical Journal* **314**, 1071–1076.

Diehl, H.S., Baker, A.B. and Cowan, D.W. 1938: Cold vaccines: an evaluation based on a controlled study. *Journal of the American Medical Association* **111**, 1168–1173.

Diehr, P., Martin, D.C., Koepsell, T., Cheadle, A., Psaty, B.M. and Wagner, E.H. 1995a: Optimal survey design for community intervention evaluations: cohort or cross-sectional? *Journal of Clinical Epidemiology* **48**, 1461–1472.

Diehr, P., Martin, D.C., Koepsell, T. and Cheadle, A. 1995b: Breaking the matches in a paired *t*-test for community interventions when the number of pairs is small. *Statistics in Medicine* **14**, 1491–1504.

Diggle, P.J., Liang, K.Y. and Zeger, S.L. 1994: *Analysis of longitudinal data*. Oxford: Oxford University Press.

Divine, G.W., Brown, J.T. and Frazier, L.M. 1992: The unit of analysis error in studies about physicians' patient care behavior. *Journal of General Internal Medicine* **7**, 623–629.

Donald, A. and Donner, A. 1987: Adjustments to the Mantel–Haenszel chi-square statistic and odds ratio variance estimator when the data are clustered. *Statistics in Medicine* **6**, 491–499.

Donner, A. 1986: A review of inference procedures for the intraclass correlation coefficient in the one-way random effects model. *International Statistical Review* **54**, 67–82.

Donner, A. 1987a: Statistical methodology for paired cluster designs. *American Journal of Epidemiology* **126**, 972–979.

Donner, A. 1987b: Odds ratio inference with dependent data: a relationship between two procedures. *Biometrika* **74**, 220.

Donner, A. 1989: Statistical methods in ophthalmology: an adjusted chi-square approach. *Biometrics* **45**, 511–605.

Donner, A. 1998: Some aspects of the design and analysis of cluster randomization trials. *Applied Statistics* **47**, 95–114.

Donner, A., Birkett, N., and Buck, C. 1981: Randomization by cluster: sample size requirements and analysis. *American Journal of Epidemiology* **114**, 906–914.

Donner, A., Brown, K.S. and Brasher, P. 1990: A methodological review of non-therapeutic intervention trials employing cluster randomization, 1979–1989. *International Journal of Epidemiology* **19**, 795–800.

Donner, A. and Donald, A. 1987: Analysis of data arising from a stratified design with the cluster as unit of randomization. *Statistics in Medicine* **6**, 43–52.

Donner, A. and Donald, A. 1988: The statistical analysis of multiple binary measurements. *Journal of Chronic Diseases* **41**, 899–905.

Donner, A., Eliasziw, M. and Klar, N. 1994: A comparison of methods for testing homogeneity of proportions in teratologic studies. *Statistics in Medicine* **13**, 1253–1264.

Donner, A. and Hauck, W. 1988: Estimation of a common odds ratio in case–control studies of familial aggregation. *Biometrics* **44**, 369–378.

Donner, A. and Hauck, W. 1989: Estimation of a common odds ratio in paired-cluster randomization designs. *Statistics in Medicine* **8**, 599–607.

Donner, A. and Klar, N. 1993: Confidence interval construction for effect measures arising from cluster randomization trials. *Journal of Clinical Epidemiology* **46**, 123–131.

Donner, A. and Klar, N. 1994a: Cluster randomization trials in epidemiology: theory and application. *Journal of Statistical Planning and Inference* **42**, 37–56.

Donner, A. and Klar, N. 1994b: Methods for comparing event rates in intervention studies when the unit of allocation is a cluster. *American Journal of Epidemiology* **140**, 279–289.

Donner, A. and Klar, N. 1996: Statistical considerations in the design and analysis of community intervention trials. *Journal of Clinical Epidemiology* **49**, 435–439.

Donner, A. and Koval, J.J. 1980: The estimation of intraclass correlation in the analysis of family data. *Biometrics* **36**, 19–25.

Duffy, S.W., South, M.C. and Day, N.E. 1992: Cluster randomization in large public health trials: the importance of antecedent data. *Statistics in Medicine* **11**, 307–316.

Duncan, C., Jones, K. and Moon, G. 1998: Context, composition and heterogeneity: using multilevel models in health research. *Social Science and Medicine* **46**, 97–117.

Dunn, G. 1994: Statistical methods for measuring outcomes. *Social Psychiatry and Psychiatric Epidemiology* **29**, 198–204.

Dunn, O.J. and Clark, V.A. 1987: *Applied statistics: analysis of variance and regression*, 2nd edn. New York: John Wiley.

Ederer, F. 1973: Shall we count numbers of eyes or numbers of subjects? *Archives of Ophthalmology* **89**, 1–2.

Editor 1937: Mathematics and medicine. *Lancet* **1**, 31.

Edwards, S.J.L., Braunholtz, D.A., Lilford, R.J. and Stevens, A.J. 1999: Ethical issues in the design and conduct of cluster randomised controlled trials. *British Medical Journal* **318**, 1407–1409.

EGRET 1990: *Epidemiological, graphics, estimation and testing package*. Seattle, WA: Statistics and Epidemiology Research Corporation.

Ellenberg, S.S. 1997: Informed consent: protection or obstacle? Some emerging issues. *Controlled Clinical Trials* **18**, 628–636.

Ellickson, P.L. 1994: Getting and keeping schools and kids for evaluation studies. *Journal of Community Psychology*. CSAP Special Issues, 102–116.

Elliott, T.E., Murray, D.M., Oken, M.M. *et al.* 1997: Improving cancer pain management in communities: main results from a randomized controlled trial. *Journal of Pain and Symptom Management* **13**, 191–203.

Ernst, E. and Herxheimer, A. 1996: The power of placebo: Let's use it to help as much as possible. *British Medical Journal* **313**, 1569–1570.

Esbensen, F.A., Deschenes, E.P., Vogel, R.E., West, J., Arboit, K. and Harris, L. 1996: Active parental consent in school-based research. *Evaluation Review* **20**, 737–753.

Everitt, B.S. 1993: *Cluster Analysis*, 3rd edn. London: Edward Arnold.

Everitt, B.S. 1995: Commentary: classification and cluster analysis. *British Medical Journal* **311**, 535–536.

Family Heart Study Group. 1994a: The British Family Heart Study: its design and methods, and prevalence of cardiovascular risk factors. *British Journal of General Practice* **44**, 62–67.

Family Heart Study Group. 1994b: Randomized controlled trial evaluating cardiovascular screening and intervention in general practice: principal results of the British Family Heart Study. *British Medical Journal* **308**, 313–320.

Farquhar, J.W. 1978: The community-based model of lifestyle intervention trials, *American Journal of Epidemiology* **108**, 103–111.

Farquhar, J.W., Maccoby, N., Wood, P.D. *et al.* 1977: Community education for cardiovascular health. *Lancet* **1**, 1192–1195.

Farr, B.M., Hendley, J.O., Kaiser, D.L. and Gwaltney, J.M. 1988: Two randomized controlled trials of virucidal nasal tissues in the prevention of natural upper respiratory infection. *American Journal of Epidemiology* **128**, 1162–1172.

Fawzi, W.W., Chalmers, T.C., Herrera, M.G. and Mosteller, F. 1993: Vitamin A supplementation and child mortality. A meta-analysis. *Journal of American Medical Association* **269**, 898–903.

Fay, M.E. and Gennings, C. 1996: Non-parametric two-sample tests for repeated ordinal responses. *Statistics in Medicine* **15**, 429–442.

Feldman, H.A. 1997: Selecting endpoint variables for a community intervention trial. *Annals of Epidemiology* Supplement 7, S78–S88.

Feldman, H.A. and McKinlay, S.M. 1994: Cohort versus cross-sectional design in large field trials: precision, sample size, and a unifying model. *Statistics in Medicine* **13**, 61–78.

Feldman, H.A., Proschan, M.A., Murray, D.M. *et al.* for REACT Study Group 1998: Statistical design of REACT (Rapid Action for Coronary Treatment) a multisite community trial with continual data collection. *Controlled Clinical Trials* **19**, 391–403.

Feng, Z. and Grizzle, J.E. 1992: Correlated binomial variates: properties of estimator of intraclass correlation and its effect on sample size calculation, *Statistics in Medicine* **11**, 1607–1614.

Ferebee, S.H., Mount, F.W., Murray, F.J. and Livesay, V.T. 1963: A controlled trial of isoniazid prophylaxis in mental institutions. *American Review of Respiratory Disease* **88**, 161–175.

Ferron, J. 1997: Moving between hierarchical modeling notations. *Journal of Educational and Behavioral Statistics* **22**, 119–123.

Festing, W.F. 1996: Are animal experiments in toxicological research the 'right' size? In Morgan, B.J.T. (ed.), *Statistics in toxicology*. Oxford: Clarendon Press, 4–11.

Fienberg, S.E. and Hinkley, D.V. (eds) 1978: *R.A. Fisher: an appreciation*. New York: Springer-Verlag.

Finney, D.J. 1947: *Probit analysis; a statistical treatment of the sigmoid response curve*. Cambridge: Cambridge University Press.

Fishbein, M. 1996: Editorial: great expectations, or do we ask too much from community-level interventions? *American Journal of Public Health* **86**, 1075–1076.

Fisher, R.A. 1926: The arrangement of field experiments. *Journal of Agriculture* **33**, 503–513.

Fisher, R.A. 1935: *The design of experiments*. Edinburgh: Oliver and Boyd.

Fisher, E.B. Jr. 1995: Editorial: the results of the COMMIT trial. *American Journal of Public Health* **85**, 159–160.

Flanders, W.D. and Kleinbaum, D.G. 1995: Basic models for disease occurrence in epidemiology. *International Journal of Epidemiology* **24**, 1–7.

Flay, B.R. 1986: Efficacy and effectiveness trials (and other phases of research) in the development of health promotion programs. *Preventive Medicine* **15**, 451–474.

Flay, B.R., Miller, T.Q., Hedeker, D. *et al.* 1995: The television, school, and family smoking prevention and cessation project. VIII, Student outcomes and mediating variables. *Preventive Medicine* **24**, 29–40.

Fleiss, J.L. 1981: *Statistical methods for rates and proportions*, 2nd edn. New York: John Wiley.

Fleiss, J.L. 1986: *The design and analysis of clinical experiments*. New York: John Wiley.

Fleiss, J.L. 1993: The statistical basis of meta-analysis. *Statistical Methods in Medical Research* **2**, 121–145.

Fleming, T.R. 1995: Interpretation of subgroup analyses in clinical trials. *Drug Information Journal* **29**, 1681S–1687S.

Fleming, T.R. and DeMets, D.L. 1996: Surrogate endpoints in clinical trials: are we being misled? *Annals of Internal Medicine* **125**, 605–613.

Fontanet, A.L., Saba, J., Chandelying, V. *et al.* 1998: Protection against sexually transmitted diseases by granting sex workers in Thailand the choice of using the male or female condom: results from a randomized controlled trial. *AIDS* **12**, 1851–1859.

Fortmann, S.P., Flora, J.A., Winkleby, M.A., Schooler, C., Taylor, C.B. and Farquhar, J.W. 1995: Community intervention trials: reflections on the Stanford five-city project experience. *American Journal Epidemiology* **142**, 576–586.

Freedman, L.S., Gail, M.H., Green, S.B. and Corle, D.K. for the COMMIT Study Group. 1997: The efficiency of the matched pairs design of the Community Intervention Trial for Smoking Cessation (COMMIT). *Controlled Clinical Trials* **18**, 131–139.

Freedman, L.S., Green, S.B. and Byar, D.P. 1990: Assessing the gain in efficiency due to matching in a community intervention study. *Statistics in Medicine* **9**, 943–952.

Freedman R, and Takeshita J.Y. 1969: *Family planning in Taiwan: an experiment in social change*. New Jersey: Princeton University Press.

Friedman, L.M., Furberg, C.D. and DeMets, D.L. 1996: *Fundamentals of clinical trials*, 3rd edn. St Louis, MO: Mosby-Year Book.

Fry, J.S. and Lee, P.N. 1988: Stratified rank tests. *Applied Statistics* **38**, 264–266.

Fuks, A., Weijer, C., Freedman, B., Shapiro, S., Skrutkowska, M. and Riaz, A. 1998: A study in contrasts: eligibility criteria in a twenty-year sample of NSABP and POG clinical trials. *Journal of Clinical Epidemiology* **51**, 69–79.

Fung, K.Y., Krewski, D., Rao, J.N. and Scott, A.J. 1994: Tests for trend in development toxicity experiments with correlated binary data. *Risk Analysis* **14**, 639–648.

Gail, M.H., Byar, D.P., Pechacek, T.F. and Corle, D.K. 1992: Aspects of statistical design for the community intervention trial for smoking cessation (COMMIT): *Controlled Clinical Trials* **13**, 6–21.

Gail, M.H., Mark, S.D., Carroll, R.J., Green, S.B. and Pee, D. 1996: On design considerations and randomization-based inference for community intervention trials. *Statistics in Medicine* **15**, 1069–1092.

Gange, S.J., DeMets, D.L. 1996: Sequential monitoring of clinical trials with correlated responses. *Biometrika* **83**, 157–167.

Gardner, M.J. and Altman, D.G. 1986: Confidence intervals rather than P-values: estimation rather than hypothesis testing. *British Medical Journal* **292**, 750–776.

Gardner, W., Mulvey, E.P. and Shaw, E.C. 1995: Regression analyses of counts and rates: Poisson, overdispersed Poisson and negative binomial models. *Psychological Bulletin* **118**, 392–404.

George, S.L. 1996: Reducing patient eligibility criteria in cancer clinical trials. *Journal of Clinical Oncology* **14**, 1364–1370.

Ghana VAST Study Team 1993: Vitamin A supplementation in northern Ghana: effects on clinic attendances, hospital admissions, and child mortality. *Lancet* **342**, 7–12.

Gilliss, C.L. and Davis, L.L. 1992: Family nursing research: precepts from paragons and peccadilloes. *Journal of Advanced Nursing* **17**, 28–33.

Gilliss, C.L., Gortner, S.R., Hauck, W.W., Shinn J.A., Sparocino, P.A. and Tompkins, C. 1993: A randomized clinical trial of nursing care for recovery from cardiac surgery. *Heart and Lung* **22**, 125–133.

Gillon, R. 1990: Ethics in health promotion and prevention of disease. *Journal of Medical Ethics* **16**, 171–172.

Gillum, R.F., Williams, P.T. and Sondik, E. 1980: Some consideration for the planning of total-community prevention trials – when is sample size adequate? *Journal of Community Health* **5**, 270–278.

Glanz, K., Rimer, B.K. and Lerman, C. 1996: Ethical issues in the design and conduct of community-based intervention studies. In Coughlin, S.S. and Beauchamp, T.L. (eds), *Ethics and epidemiology*. Oxford: Oxford University Press, Ch. 8.

Glasgow, R.E., Lichtenstein, E., Wilder, D., Hall, R., McRae, S.G. and Liberty, B. 1995a: The tribal tobacco policy project: working with Northwest Indian tribes on smoking policies. *Preventive Medicine* **24**, 434–440.

Glasgow, R.E., Terborg, J.R., Hollis, J.F., Severson, H.H. and Boles, S.M. 1995b: Take Heart: results from the initial phase of a work-site wellness program. *American Journal of Public Health* **85**, 209–216.

Glass, G.V. and Stanley, J.C. 1970: *Statistical methods in education and psychology*. Englewood Cliffs, NJ: Prentice-Hall.

Glynn, R.J., Rosner, B. 1992: Accounting for the correlation between fellow eyes in regression analysis. *Archives of Ophthalmology* **110**, 381–387.

Goldstein, H. 1995: *Multi-level statistical models*, 2nd edn. London: Arnold.

Goldstein, H., Rasbah, J., Plewis, I. *et al.* 1998: *A user's guide to MlwiN*. London, UK: Multilevel Models Project, Institute of Education, University of London.

Graham, J.W., Flay, B.R., Johnson, C.A., Hansen, W.B. and Collins, L.M. 1984: A multiattribute utility measurement approach to the use of random assignment with small number of aggregated units. *Evaluation Review* **8**, 247–260.

Grant, A., Valentin, L., Elbourne, D. and Alexander, S. 1989: Routine formal fetal movement counting and risk of antepartum late death in normally formed singletons. *Lancet* **2**, 345–349.

Gray-Donald, K., Kramer, M.S., Munday, S. and Leduc, D.C. 1985: Effect of formula supplementation in the hospital on the duration of breast-feeding: a controlled clinical trials. *Pediatrics* **76**, 514–518.

Green, S.B. 1997: The advantages of community-randomized trials for evaluating lifestyle modification. *Controlled Clinical Trials* **18**, 506–513.

Greenhalgh, T. 1997: The Medline database. *British Medical Journal* **315**, 180–183.

Greenwald, P. and Kelloff, G.J. 1996: The role of chemoprevention in cancer control, In Stewart B.W., McGregor, D. and Kleihues, P. (eds), *Principles of chemoprevention.* IARC Scientific Publications No. 139. Lyon: International Agency for Research on Cancer, 13–22.

Grosskurth, H., Mosha, F., Todd, J. *et al.* 1995: Impact of improved treatment of sexually transmitted diseases on HIV infection in rural Tanzania: randomized controlled trial. *Lancet* **346**, 530–536.

Grossman, D.C., Neckerman, H.J., Koepsell, T.D. *et al.* 1997: Effectiveness of a violence prevention curriculum among children in elementary school. A randomized controlled trial. *Journal of the American Medical Association* **277**, 1605–1611.

Groves, F.D., Zavala, D.E. and Correa, P. 1987: Variation in international cancer mortality: factor and cluster analysis. *International Journal of Epidemiology* **16**, 501–508.

Gulliford, M.C., Ukoumunne, O.C. and Chinn, S. 1999: Components of variance and intraclass correlations for the design of community-based surveys and intervention studies, Data from the Health Survey for England 1994. *American Journal of Epidemiology* **149**, 876–883.

Gyorkos, T.W., Frappier-Davignon, L., MacLean, J.D. and Viens, P. 1989: Effect of screening and treatment on imported intestinal parasite infections: results from a randomized controlled trial. *American Journal of Epidemiology* **129**, 753–761.

Hacking, I. 1988: Telepathy: origins of randomization in experimental design. *ISIS* **79**, 427–451.

Haggerty, P.A., Muladi, K., Kirkwood, B.R., Ashworth, A. and Manunebo, M. 1994: Community-based hygiene education to reduce diarrhoeal disease in rural Zaire: impact of the intervention on diarrhoeal morbidity. *International Journal of Epidemiology* **23**, 1050–1059.

Halperin, M., Cornfield, J. and Mitchell, S.C. 1973: Effect of diet on coronary-heart-disease mortality. *Lancet* **2**, 438–439.

Hand, D.J., 1996: Statistics and the theory of measurement. *Journal of the Royal Statistical Society* **159**, 445–492.

Hannan, P.J., Murray, D.M., Jacobs, D.R. and McGovern, P.G. 1994: Parameters to aid in the design and analysis of community trials: intraclass correlations from Minnesota Heart Health Program. *Epidemiology* **5**, 88–95.

Hannan, P.J. and Murray, D.M. 1996: Gauss or Bernoulli? A Monte Carlo comparison of the performance of the linear mixed model and the logistic mixed model analyses in simulated community trials with a dichotomous outcome variable at the individual level. *Evaluation Review* **20**, 338–352.

Hansen, M.H. and Hurwitz, W.N. 1942: Relative efficiencies of various sampling units in population inquiries. *Journal of the American Statistical Association* **37**, 89–94.

Hansen, M.H., Hurwitz, W.N. and Madow, W.G. 1953: *Sample survey methods and theory, vol. 1, Methods and applications.* New York: John Wiley.

Hardcastle, J.D., Chamberlain, J.O., Robinson, M.H.E. *et al.* 1996: Randomised controlled trial of faecal-occult-blood screening for colorectal cancer, *Lancet* **348**, 1472–1477.

Harrington, K.F., Binkley, D., Reynolds, K.D. *et al.* 1997: Recruitment issues in school-based research: lessons learned from the High 5 Alabama Project. *Journal of School Health* **67**, 415–421.

Harris, J.E. 1985: Macroexperiments versus microexperiments for health policy. In Hausman, J.A. and Wise, D.A. (eds), *Social experimentation*. Chicago: University of Chicago Press, Ch. 4.

Haseman, J.K. and Hogan, M.D. 1975: Selection of the experimental unit in teratology studies. *Teratology* **12**, 165–171.

Hauck, W.W., Anderson, S. and Marcus, S.M. 1998: Should we adjust for covariates in nonlinear regression analyses of randomized trials? *Controlled Clinical Trials* **19**, 249–256.

Hayes, R. 1998: Design of human immunodeficiency virus intervention trials in developing countries. *Journal of the Royal Statistical Society, Series A* **161**, 251–263.

Hayes, R.J. and Bennett, S. 1999: Simple sample size calculation for cluster-randomized trials. *International Journal of Epidemiology* **28**, 319–326.

Hayes, R., Mosha, F., Nicoll, A. *et al.* 1995: A community trial of the impact of improved sexually transmitted disease treatment on the HIV epidemic in rural Tanzania: 1. Design. *AIDS* **9**, 919–926.

Hedeker, D. and Gibbons, R.D. 1996: MIXOR: a computer program for mixed-effects ordinal regression analysis. *Computer Methods and Programs in Biomedicine* **49**, 157–176.

Hedeker, D., Gibbons, R.D. and Flay, B.R. 1994b: Random-effects regression models for clustered data with an example from smoking prevention research. *Journal of Consulting and Clinical Psychology* **62**, 757–765.

Hedeker, D., McMahon, S.D., Jason, L.A. and Salina, D. 1994a: Analysis of clustered data in community psychology: with an example from a worksite smoking cessation project. *American Journal of Community Psychology* **22**, 595–615.

Heeren, T. and D'Agostino, R. 1987: Robustness of the two-independent samples *t*-test when applied to ordinal scaled data. *Statistics in Medicine* **6**, 79–90.

Heitjan, D.F. 1997: Annotation: what can be done about missing data? Approaches to imputation. *American Journal of Public Health* **87**, 548–550.

Henderson, M.M. and Meinert, C.L. 1975: A plea for a discipline of health and medical evaluation. *International Journal of Epidemiology* **4**, 11–23.

Henderson, W.G., Moritz, T., Goldman, S. *et al.* 1988: The statistical analysis of graft patency data in a clinical trial of antiplatelet agents following coronary artery bypass grafting. *Controlled Clinical Trials* **9**, 189–205.

Herrera, M.G., Nestel, P., El Amin, A., Fawzi, W.W., Muhammad, K.A. and Weld, L.1992: Vitamin A supplementation and child survival. *Lancet* **340**, 267–271.

Hill, A.B. 1990: Memories of the British streptomycin trial in tuberculosis. The first randomized clinical trial. *Controlled Clinical Trials*, 11, 77–79.

Hilton, E.T. and Lumsdaine, A.A. 1975: Field trial designs in gauging the impact of fertility planning programs. In Bennett, C.A. and Lumsdaine, A.A. (eds), *Evaluation and experiment*. New York: Academic Press, 319–408.

Hinshaw, H.C. and Feldman, W.H. 1944: Evaluation of chemotherapeutic agents in clinical tuberculosis. *American Review of Tuberculosis* **50**, 202–213.

Holt, D. 1989: Panel conditioning: discussion, In Kasprzyk, D., Duncan, G.J., Kalton, G. and Singh, M.P. (eds), *Panel surveys*. New York: John Wiley, 340–347

Hopkins, K.D. 1982: The unit of analysis: group means versus individual observations. *American Educational Research Journal* **19**, 5–18.

Horwitz, O. and Magnus, K. 1974: Epidemiologic evaluation of chemoprophylaxis against tuberculosis. *American Journal of Epidemiology* **99**, 333–342.

Hosmer, D.W. and Lemeshow, S. 1999: *Applied survival analysis*. New York: John Wiley.

Houston, C.S. 1991: *R.G. Ferguson: crusader against tuberculosis*. Toronto: Hannah Institute and Dundurn Press.

Howard-Jones, N. 1982: Human experimentation in historical and ethical perspectives. *Social Science and Medicine* **16**, 1429–1448.

Howard-Pitney, B., Winkleby, M.A., Albright, C.L., Bruce, B. and Fortmann, S.P. 1997: The Stanford nutrition action program: a dietary fat intervention for low-literacy adults. *American Journal of Public Health* **87**, 1971–1976.

Hsieh, F.Y. 1988: Sample size formulae for intervention studies with the cluster as unit of randomization. *Statistics in Medicine* **8**, 1195–1201.

Huber, P.J. 1967: The behavior of maximum likelihood estimates under nonstandard conditions, In Lecam, L.M. and Neyman, J. (eds), *Proceedings of the Fifth Berkeley Symposium in mathematical statistics and probability*. Berkeley, CA: University of California Press, 221–233.

Hulley, S.B. 1978: Symposium on CHD prevention trials: design issues in testing life style interventions; introduction. *American Journal of Epidemiology* **108**, 85–86.

Hunt, J.R. and White, E. 1998: Retaining and tracking cohort study members. *Epidemiologic Reviews* **20**, 57–70.

Imrey, P.B. 1986: Considerations in the statistical analysis of clinical trials in periodontitis. *Journal of Clinical Periodontology* **13**, 517–528.

Imrey, P.B. and Chilton, N.W. 1992: Design and analytic concepts for periodontal clinical trials. *Journal of Periodontology* **63**, 1124–1140.

Jason, L.A., Jayaraj, S., Blitz, C.C., Michaels, M.H. and Klett, L.E. 1990: Incentives and competition in a worksite smoking cessation intervention. *American Journal of Public Health* **80**, 205–206.

Jemmott, J.B. III, Jemmott, L.S., and Fong, G.T. 1998: Abstinence and safer sex HIV risk reduction interventions. *Journal of the American Medical Association* **279**, 1529–1536.

Joffe, M.M. and Rosenbaum, P.R. 1999: Invited commentary: propensity scores. *American Journal of Epidemiology* **150**, 327–333.

Jones, B., Jarvis, P., Lewis, J.A. and Ebbutt, A.F. 1996: Trials to assess equivalence: the importance of rigorous methods. *British Medical Journal* **313**, 36–39.

Jooste, P.L., Yach, D., Steenkamp, H.J., Botha, J.L. and Rossouw, J.E. 1990: Drop-out and newcomer bias in a community cardiovascular follow-up study. *International Journal of Epidemiology* **19**, 284–289.

Katz, J., Carey, V.J., Zeger, S.L. and Sommer, A. 1993a: Estimation of design effects and diarrhea clustering within households and villages. *American Journal of Epidemiology* **138**, 994–1006

Katz, J. and Zeger, S.L. 1994: Estimation of design effects in cluster surveys. *Annals of Epidemiology* **4**, 295–301.

Katz, J., Zeger, S.L., West, K.P. Jr, Tielsch, J.M. and Sommer, A. 1993b: Clustering of xerophthalmia within households and villages. *International Journal of Epidemiology* **22**, 709–715.

Kegeles, S.M., Hays, R.B. and Coates, T.J. 1996: The Mpowerment project: a community-level HIV prevention intervention for young gay men. *American Journal of Public Health* **86**, 1129–1136.

Kelder, S.H., Jacobs, D.R. Jr, Jeffery, R.W., McGovern, P.G. and Forster, J.L. 1993: The worksite component of variance: design effects and the Healthy Worker Project. *Health Education Research* **8**, 555–566.

Kelsey, J.L., Whittemore, A.S., Evans, A.S. and Thompson, D.L. 1996: *Methods in observational epidemiology*, 2nd edn. New York: Oxford University Press.

Kerry, S. and Bland, J.M. 1998: Analysis of a trial randomized in clusters. *British Medical Journal* **316**, 549.

Kerry, S. and Bland, J.M. 1998: Statistics notes: the intracluster correlation in cluster randomization. *British Medical Journal* **316**, 1455.

Keselman, H.J., Algina, J., Kowalchuk, R.K. and Wolfinger, R.D. 1998: A comparison of two approaches for selecting covariance structures in the analysis of repeated measures. *Communications in Statistics – Simulation* **27**, 591–604.

Kilgore, E.S. 1920: Relation of quantitative methods to the advance of medical science. *Journal of American Medical Association* **75**, 86–89.

Kirkwood, B.R., Cousens, S.N., Victora, C.G. and de Zoysa, I. 1997: Issues in the design and interpretation of studies to evaluate the impact of community-based interventions. *Tropical Medicine and International Health* **2**, 1022–1029.

Kirkwood, B.R. and Morrow, R.H. 1989: Community-based intervention trials. *Journal of Biosocial Sciences*, Supplement 10, 79–86.

Kish, L. 1965: *Survey sampling*. New York: John Wiley.

Klar, N. 1996: Stratified analysis of correlated binary outcome: a comparison of model dependent and robust tests of significance. *Communications in Statistics – Theory and Methods* **25**, 2431–2458.

Klar, N. and Donner, A. 1997: The merits of matching in community intervention trials. *Statistics in Medicine* **16**, 1753–1764.

Klar, N., Gyorkos, T. and Donner, A. 1995: Cluster randomization trials in tropical medicine: a case study. *Transactions of the Royal Society of Tropical Medicine and Hygiene* **89**, 454–459.

Kleinbaum, D.G. 1996: *Survival analysis, a self-learning text*. New York: Springer-Verlag.

Koepsell, T.D. 1998: Epidemiologic issues in the design of community intervention trials. In Brownson, R.C. and Petitti, D.B. (eds), *Applied epidemiology: theory to practice*. New York: Oxford University Press, 177–211.

Koepsell, T.D., Martin, D.C., Diehr, P.H. *et al.* 1991: Data analysis and sample size issues in evaluations of community-based health promotion and disease prevention programs: a mixed-model analysis of variance approach. *Journal of Clinical Epidemiology* **44**, 701–713.

Koepsell, T.D., Wagner, E.H., Cheadle, A.C. *et al.* 1992: Selected methodological issues in evaluating community-based health promotion and disease prevention programs. *Annual Review of Public Health* **13**, 31–57.

Korn, E.L. 1984: The paired *t*-test. *Applied Statistics* **33**, 230–231.

Kramer, M.S. 1988: *Clinical epidemiology and biostatistics: a primer for clinical investigators and decision-makers*. New York: Springer-Verlag.

Kreft, I.G.G., de Leeuw, J. and van der Leeden, R. 1994: Review of five multilevel analysis programs: BMDP-5V, GENMOD, HLM, ML3, VARCL. *The American Statistician* **48**, 324–335.

Kreft, I.G.G. 1998: An illustration of item homogeneity scaling and multilevel analysis techniques in the evaluation of drug prevention programs. *Evaluation Review* **22**, 46–77.

Krewski, D., Leroux, B.G. and Zhu, Y. 1996: Statistical analysis of toxicological experiments on carcinogenicity, mutagenicity, and developmental toxicity. In Armitage, P. and David, H.A. (eds), *Advances in biometry*. New York: John Wiley, 423–448.

Kronborg, O., Fenger, C., Olsen, J., Jorgensen, O.D., and Sondergaard, O. 1996: Randomised study of screening for colorectal cancer with faecal-occult-blood test. *Lancet* **348**, 1467–1471.

Kruskal, W.H. 1957: Historical notes on the Wilcoxon unpaired two-sample test. *Journal of the American Statistical Association* **52**, 356–360.

Kvalem, I.L., Sundet, J.M., Rivo, K.I., Eilertsen, D.E. and Bakketeig, L.S. 1996: The effect of sex education on adolescents' use of condoms: applying the Solomon four-group design. *Health Education Quarterly* **23**, 34–47.

Lachin, J.M. 1981: Introduction to sample size determination and power analysis for clinical trials. *Controlled Clinical Trials* **2**, 93–113.

Lachin, J.M. and Bautista, O.M. 1995: Stratified-adjusted versus unstratified assessment of sample size and power for analyses of proportions. In Thall, P.F. (ed.), *Recent advances in clinical trial design and analysis*. Boston: Kluwer Academic, 203–224.

LaPrelle, J., Bauman, K.E. and Koch, G.C. 1992: High intercommunity variation in adolescent cigarette smoking in a 10-community field experiment. *Evaluation Review* **16**, 115–130.

Lasater, T.M., Becker, D.M., Hill, M.N. and Gans, K.M. 1997: Synthesis of findings and issues from religious-based cardiovascular disease prevention trials. *Annals of Epidemiology* **7**, S46–S53.

Last, J.M. 1991: Epidemiology and Ethics. In Bankowski, Z., Bryant, J.H. and Last, J.M. (eds), *Ethics and epidemiology: international guidelines. Proceedings of the XXVth CIOMS Conference*. Geneva: CIOMS, 14–28.

Last, J.M. (ed.) 1995: *A dictionary of epidemiology*, 3rd edn. Oxford: Oxford University Press.

Lavange, L.M., Keyes, L.L., Koch, G.G. and Margolis, P.A. 1994: Application of sample survey methods for modelling ratios to incidence densities. *Statistics in Medicine* **13**, 343–355.

Le, C.T. and Lindgren, B.R. 1996: Duration of ventilating tubes: a test for comparing two clustered samples of censored data. *Biometrics* **52**, 328–334.

Lehmann, E.L. 1975: *Nonparametrics. Statistical methods based on ranks*. Oakland, CA: Holden-Day.

Levy, P.S. and Lemeshow, S. 1980: *Sampling for Health Professionals*. Belmont, CA: Lifetime Learning Publications.

Liang, K. 1985: Odds ratio inference with dependent data. *Biometrika* **72**, 678–682.

Liang, K.Y., Beaty, T.H. and Cohen, B.H, 1986: Application of odds ratio regression models for assessing familial aggregation from case-control studies. *American Journal of Epidemiology* **124**, 678–683.

Liang, K-Y. and Zeger, S.L. 1986: Longitudinal data analysis using generalized linear models. *Biometrika* **73**, 13–22.

Lin, D.Y. 1994: Cox regression analysis of multivariate failure time data: the marginal approach. *Statistics in Medicine* **13**, 2233–2247.

Lindquist, E.F. 1940: *Statistical analysis in educational research*. Boston: Houghton Mifflin.

Littell, R.C., Milliken, G.A., Stroup, W.W. and Wolfinger, R.D. 1996: *SAS system for mixed models*. Cary, NC: SAS Institute Inc.

Longford, N. 1993: *Random coefficient models*. Oxford: Clarendon Press.

Lubsen, J. and Pocock, S.J. 1994: Factorial trials in cardiology: pros and cons. *European Heart Journal* **15**, 585–588.

Luepker, R.V., Perry, C.L., McKinlay, S.M. *et al.* for the CATCH Collaborative Group 1996: Outcomes of a field trial to improve children's dietary patterns and physical activity. *Journal of the American Medical Association* **275**, 768–776.

Lurie, P., Bishaw, M., Chesney, M.A. *et al.* 1994: Ethical, behavioral and social aspects of HIV vaccine trials in developing countries. *Journal of the American Medical Association* **271**, 295–301.

Macdonald, L.A., Sackett, D.L., Haynes, R.B. and Taylor, D.W. 1984: Labelling in hypertension: a review of the behavioural and psychological consequences, *Journal of Chronic Diseases* **37**, 933–942.

MacMahon, B. and Pugh, T.F. 1970: *Epidemiology, principles and methods*. Boston, MA: Little, Brown.

Mainland, D. 1934: Chance and the blood count. *Canadian Medical Association Journal* **30**, 656–658.

Mainland, D. 1936: Problems of chance in clinical work. *British Medical Journal* **2**, 221–224.

Mainland, D. 1952: *Elementary medical statistics; the principles of quantitative medicine*. Philadelphia: W.B. Saunders.

Mantel, N. and Haenszel, W. 1959: Statistical aspects of the analysis of data from retrospective studies of disease. *Journal of the National Cancer Institute* **22**, 719–748.

Marbiah, N.T., Petersen, E., David, K., Magbity, E., Lines, J. and Bradley, D.J. 1998: A controlled trial of lambda-cyhalothrin-impregnated bed nets and/or dapsone/pyrimethamine for malaria control in Sierra Leone. *American Journal Tropical Medicine and Hygiene* **58**, 1–6.

Maritz, J.S. and Jarrett, R.G., 1983: The use of statistics to examine the association between fluoride in drinking water and cancer death rates. *Applied Statistics* **32**, 97–101.

Marks, H.M. 1997: *The progress of experiment, science and therapeutic reform in the United States, 1900–1990*. Cambridge: Cambridge University Press.

Marshall, K.G. 1996: Prevention. How much harm? How much benefit? 4. The ethics of informed consent for preventive screening programs. *Canadian Medical Association Journal* **155**, 377–383.

Marteau, T.M., Kinmonth, A.L., Thompson, S. and Pyke, S. 1996: The psychological impact of cardiovascular screening and intervention in primary care: a problem of false reassurance? *British Journal of General Practice* **46**, 577–582.

Martin, D.C., Diehr, P., Perrin, E.B. and Koepsell, T.D. 1993: The effect of matching on the power of randomized community intervention studies. *Statistics in Medicine* **12**, 329–338.

Marubini, E., Correa Leite, M.L. and Milani, S. 1988: Analysis of dichotomous response variables in teratology. *Biometrical Journal* **30**, 965–974.

Matthews, J.N.S., Altman, D.G., Campbell, M.J. and Royston, P. 1990: Analysis of serial measurements in medical research. *British Medical Journal* **300**, 230–235.

Matthews, J.R. 1995: *Quantification and the quest for medical certainty*. Princeton, NJ: Princeton University Press.

Mayer, J.A., Slymen, D.J., Eckhardt, L. *et al.* 1998: Skin cancer prevention counseling by pharmacists: specific outcomes of an intervention trial. *Cancer Detection & Prevention* **22**, 367–375.

Mayne, S.T., Handelman, G.J. and Beecher, G. 1996: Beta-carotene and lung cancer promotion in heavy smokers – a plausible relationship. *Journal of the National Cancer Institute* **88**, 1513–1515.

McArdle, C.S. and Hole, D. 1991: Impact of variability among surgeons on postoperative morbidity and mortality and ultimate survival. *British Medical Journal* **302**, 1501–1505.

McCall, W.A. 1923: *How to experiment in education*. New York: Macmillan.

McFadden E. 1997: *Management of data in clinical trials*. New York: John Wiley.

McKinlay, S.M. 1994: Cost-efficient designs of cluster unit trials. *Preventive Medicine* **23**, 606–611.

McKinlay, S.M., Stone, E.J. and Zucker, D.M. 1989: Research design and analysis issues. *Health Education Quarterly* **16**, 307–313.

McLean, S. 1997: Commentary: no consent means not treating the patient with respect. *British Medical Journal* **314**, 1076.

McNemar, Q. 1940: Book review of Lindquist EF. Statistical analysis in educational research. *Psychological Bulletin* **37**, 746–748.

Medical Research Council 1948: Streptomycin treatment of pulmonary tuberculosis. *British Medical Journal* **2**, 769–782.

Mehta, C. and Patel, N. 1997: *Proc-StatXact for SAS Users, statistical software for exact nonparametric inference user manual*. Cambridge, MA: CYTEL Software Corporation.

Menzies, R., Tamblyn, R., Farant, J.P., Hanley, J., Nunes, F. and Tamblyn, R. 1993: The effect of varying levels of outdoor-air supply on the symptoms of sick building syndrome. *New England Journal of Medicine* **328**, 821–827.

Mian, I.U. and Shoukri, M.M. 1997: Statistical analysis of intraclass correlations from multiple samples with applications to arterial blood pressure data. *Statistics in Medicine* **16**, 1497–1514.

Mickey, R.M. and Goodwin, G.D. 1993: The magnitude and variability of design effects for community intervention trials. *American Journal of Epidemiology* **137**, 9–18.

Mickey, R.M., Goodwin, G.D. and Costanza, M.C. 1991: Estimation of the design effect in community intervention studies. *Statistics in Medicine* **10**, 53–64.

Miller, A.B. 1996: Fundamental issues in screening for cancer. In Schottendeld, D. and Fraumeni, J.F. Jr (eds), *Cancer epidemiology and control*, 2nd edn. Oxford: Oxford University Press. Ch. 66.

Miller, R.G. 1997: *Beyond ANOVA. Basics of applied statistics*. New York: Chapman and Hall.

Miller, P. and Plant, M. 1996: Drinking, smoking, and illicit drug use among 15 and 16 year olds in the United Kingdom. *British Medical Journal* **313**, 394–397.

Moher, D., Dulberg, C.S. and Wells, G.A. 1994: Statistical power, sample size and their reporting in randomized controlled trials. *Journal of the American Medical Association* **272**, 122–124.

Moore, D.F. and Tsiatis, A. 1991: Robust estimation of the variance in moment methods for extra-binomial and extra-Poisson variation. *Biometrics* **47**, 383–401.

Morgenstern, H. 1998: Ecologic studies. In Rothman, K.J. and Greenland, S. (eds), *Modern epidemiology*, 2nd edn. Philadelphia. PA: Lippincott-Raven. Ch. 22.

Morris, C.N., Norton, E.C. and Zhou, X.H. 1994: Parametric duration analysis of nursing home usage. In Lange, N., Ryan, L., Billard, L., Brillinger, D., Conquest, L. and Greenhouse, J. (eds), *Case studies in biometry*. New York: John Wiley. Ch. 12.

Morris, R.W. 1993: Bilateral procedures in randomised controlled trials. *Journal of Bone and Joint Surgery* (*Br*) **75-B**, 657–676.

Morrison, T.C., Wahlgren, D.R., Hovell, M.F. *et al.* 1997: Tracking and follow-up of 16,915 adolescents: minimizing attrition bias. *Controlled Clinical Trials* **18**, 383–396.

Morrow, A.L., Guerrero, M.L., Shults, J. *et al.* 1999: Efficacy of home-based peer counselling to promote exclusive breastfeeding: a randomised controlled trial. *Lancet* **353**, 1226–1231.

Moser, C.A. and Kalton, G. 1972: *Survey methods in social investigation*, 2nd edn. New York: Basic Books.

Mudde, A.N., de Vries, H. and Dolders, M.G.T. 1995: Evaluation of a Dutch community-based smoking cessation intervention. *Preventive Medicine* **24**, 61–70.

Murray, D.M. 1998: *Design and analysis of community trials*. Oxford: Oxford University Press.

Murray, D.M. 1997: Design and analysis of group-randomized trials: a review of recent developments. *Annals of Epidemiology* **7**(Supplement), S69–S77.

Murray, D.M. and Hannan, P.J. 1990: Planning for the appropriate analysis in school-based drug-use prevention studies. *Journal of Consulting and Clinical Psychology* **58**, 458–468.

Murray, D.M., Hannan, P.J., Wolfinger, R.D., Baker, W.L. and Dwyeer, J.H. 1998: Analysis of data from group-randomized trials with repeat observations on the same groups. *Statistics in Medicine* **17**, 1581–1600.

Murray, D.M., Hannan, P.J. and Zucker, D.M. 1989: Analysis issues in school-based health promotion studies. *Health Education Quarterly* **16**, 315–320.

Murray, D.M., Perry, C.L., Griffin, G. *et al.* 1992: Results from a statewide approach to adolescent tobacco use prevention. *Preventive Medicine* **21**, 449–472.

Murray, D.M., Rooney, B.L., Hannan, P.J. *et al.* 1994: Intraclass correlation among common measures of adolescent smoking: estimates, correlates, and applications in smoking prevention studies. *American Journal of Epidemiology* **140**, 1038–1050.

Murray, D.M. and Short, B. 1995: Intraclass correlation among measures related to alcohol use by young adults: estimates, correlates and applications in intervention studies. *Journal of Studies on Alcohol* **56**, 681–694.

Murray, D.M. and Short, B.J. 1997: Intraclass correlation among measures related to tobacco use by adolescents: estimates, correlates, and applications in intervention studies. *Addictive Behaviors* **22**, 1–12.

Murray, D.M. and Wolfinger, R.D. 1994: Analysis issues in the evaluation of community trials: progress toward solutions in STAT/STAT MIXED. *Journal of Community Psychology*, CSAP Special Issue, 140–154.

Murray, J.P., Stam, A. and Lastovicka, J.L. 1993: Evaluating an anti-drinking and driving advertising campaign with a sample-survey and time series intervention analysis. *Journal of the American Statistical Association* **88**, 50–56.

Neuhaus, J.M. 1992: Statistical methods for longitudinal and clustered designs with binary responses. *Statistical Methods in Medical Research* **1**, 249–273.

Neuhaus, J.M. and Kalbfleisch, J.D. 1998: Between- and within-cluster covariate effects in the analysis of clustered data. *Biometrics* **54**, 638–645.

Neuhaus, J.M. and Segal, M.R. 1993: Design effects for binary regression models fitted to dependent data. *Statistics in Medicine* **12**, 1259–1268.

Neuhauser, D.B. and Green, S.B. 1998: Efficient clinical research. *Controlled Clinical Trials* **19**, 427–429.

Newhouse, J.P. and the Insurance Experiment Group. 1993: *Free for all?: lessons from the Rand Health Insurance Experiment: a RAND study*. Cambridge, MA: Harvard University Press.

Neyman, J. 1934: On the two different aspects of the representative method: the method of stratified sampling and the method of purposive selection. *Journal of the Royal Statistical Society* **97**, 558–606.

Nystrom, L., Rutqvist, L.R., Wall, S. *et al.* 1993: Breast cancer screening with mammography: overview of Swedish randomised trials. *Lancet* **341**, 973–978.

O'Brien, P.C. and Fleming, T.R. 1979: A multiple testing procedure for clinical trials. *Biometrics* **34**, 549–556.

Oakeshott, P., Kerry, S.M. and Williams, J.E. 1994: Randomized controlled trial of the effect of the Royal College of Radiologists' referral for radiographic examination. *British Journal of General Practice* **44**, 197–200.

Oakley, A. 1998: Experimentation and social interventions: a forgotten but important history. *British Medical Journal* **317**, 1239–1242.

Office for Protection from Research Risks. 1994: *Protection of Human Subjects, Title 45, Code of Federal Regulations, Part 46*. Bethesda, MD: Department of Health and Human Services NIH.

Paci, E. and Alexander, F.E. 1997: Study design of randomized controlled clinical trials of breast screening. *Journal of the National Cancer Institute Monographs* **22**, 21–25.

Pack, S.E. 1986: Hypothesis testing for proportions with overdispersion. *Biometrics* **42**, 967–972.

Palmer, R.H., Louis, T.A., Hsu, L.N. *et al.* 1985: A randomized controlled trial of quality assurance in sixteen ambulatory care practices. *Medical Care* **23**, 751–770.

Payment, P., Richardson, L., Siemiatycki, J., Dewar, R., Edwardes, M. and Franco, E. 1991: A randomized trial to evaluate the risk of gastrointestinal disease due to consumption of drinking water meeting microbiological standards. *American Journal of Public Health* **81**, 703–708.

Peacock, J.L., Bland, J.M. and Anderson, J.H. 1995: Preterm delivery: effects of socioeconomic factors, psychological stress, smoking, alcohol, and caffeine. *British Medical Journal* **311**, 531–535.

Pearson, E.S. 1966: The Neyman–Pearson story: 1926–34. In David, F.M. (ed.), *Research papers in statistics; Festschrift for J. Neyman*. New York: John Wiley.

Pearson, K. 1904: Report on certain enteric fever inoculation statistics, *British Medical Journal* **2**, 1243–1246.

Peirce, C.S. and Jastrow, J. 1885: On small differences of sensation. *Memoirs of the National Academy of Sciences for 1884* **3**, 75–83.

Piantadosi, S. 1997: *Clinical trials: a methodologic perspective*. New York: John Wiley.

Pinol, A., Bergel, E., Chaisiri, K., Diaz, E., Gandeh, M. for the WHO Antenatal Care Trial Research Group. 1998: Managing data for a randomised controlled clinical, trial: experience from the WHO Antenatal Care Trial. *Paediatric and Perinatal Epidemiology* **12**(Suppl. 2), 142–155.

Pocock, S.J. 1983: *Clinical trials. a practical approach*. New York: John Wiley.

Pocock, S.J. 1996: Clinical Trials: A Statistician's Perspective, In Armitage, P. and David, H.A. (eds), *Advances in biometry*. New York: John Wiley, Ch. 20.

Pollock, T.M. 1966: *Trials of prophylactic agents for the control of communicable diseases; a guide to their organization and evaluation*. Monograph Series No. 52. Geneva: WHO.

Pradhan, E.K., Katz, J., LeClerq, S.C. and West, K.P. Jr 1994: Data management for large community trials in Nepal. *Controlled Clinical Trials* **15**, 220–234.

Proschan, M.A. 1996: On the distribution of the unpaired t-statistic with paired data. *Statistics in Medicine* **15**, 1059–1063.

Rao, J.N.K. and Bellhouse, D.R. 1990: History and development of the theoretical foundations of survey based estimation and analysis. *Survey Methodology* **16**, 3–29.

Rao, J.N.K. and Scott, A.J. 1992: A simple method for the analysis of clustered binary data. *Biometrics* **48**, 577–585.

Rao, J.N.K. and Scott, A.J. 1999: A simple method for analysing overdispersion in clustered Poisson data. *Statistics in Medicine* **18**, 1373–1385.

Rao, J.N.K. and Thomas, D.R. 1988: The analysis of cross-classified categorical data from complex sample surveys. *Sociological Methodology* **18**, 213–269.

Raudenbush, S.W. 1993: Hierarchical linear models and experimental design. In Edwards, L.K. (ed.), *Applied analysis of variance in behavioral science*. New York: Marcel Dekker, Ch. 13.

Raudenbush, S.W. 1997: Statistical analysis and optimal design for cluster randomization trials. *Psychological Methods* **2**, 173–185.

Ray, W.A., Taylor, J.A., Meador, K.G. *et al.* 1997: A randomized trial of a consultation service to reduce falls in nursing homes. *Journal of the American Medical Association* **278**, 557–562.

Rhee, S.O., Luke, R.D. and Culverwell, M.B. 1980: Influence of client/colleague dependence on physician performance in patient care. *Medical Care* **18**, 829–839.

Rice, N. and Leyland, A. 1996: Multilevel models: applications to health data. *Journal of Health Services Research and Policy* **3**, 154–164.

Ridout, M.S., Demètrio, C.G.B. and Firth, D. 1999: Estimating intraclass correlation for binary data. *Biometrics* **55**, 137–148.

Rooney, B.L. and Murray, D.L. 1996: A meta-analysis of smoking prevention programs after adjustment for errors in the unit of analysis. *Health Education Quarterly* **23**, 48–64.

Rose, G. 1970: A proposed trial of heart disease prevention in industry. *Transactions of the Society of Occupational Medicine* **20**, 109–111.

Rosner, B. 1984: Multivariate methods in ophthalmology with application to other paired-data situations. *Biometrics* **40**, 1025–1035.

Rosner, B. 1995: *Fundamentals of biostatistics*, 4th edn. Belmont, CA: Wadsworth.

Rosner, B, and Hennekens, C.H. 1978: Analytic methods in matched pair epidemiological studies. *International Journal of Epidemiology* **7**, 367–372.

Rothman, K.J. 1996: Placebo mania. As medical knowledge accumulates, the number of placebo trials should fall. *British Medical Journal* **313**, 3–4.

SAS Institute Inc. 1997: *SAS/STAT Software: changes and enhancements through release 6.12*. Cary, NC: SAS Institute.

Sanson-Fisher, R., Redman, S., Hancock, L. *et al.* 1996: Developing methodologies for evaluating community-wide health promotion. *Health Promotion International* **11**, 227–236.

Schain, W.S. 1994: Barriers to clinical trials. Part II: knowledge and attitudes of potential participants. *Cancer* **74** (Suppl.) 2666–2671.

Schlegel, R.P. 1977: Some methodological procedures for the evaluation of educational programs for prevention of adolescent alcohol use and abuse. *Evaluation Quarterly* **1**, 657–672.

Schwartz, D., Flamant, R. and Lellouch, J. 1980: *Clinical trials*. New York: Academic Press.

Scott, A.J. and Holt, D. 1982: The effect of two-stage sampling on ordinary least squares methods. *Journal of American Statistical Association* **77**, 848–854.

Searle, S.R., Casella, G. and McCulloch, C.E. 1992: *Variance components*. New York: John Wiley.

Segal, M.R. and Neuhaus, J.M. 1993: Robust inference for multivariate survival data. *Statistics in Medicine* **12**, 1019–1031.

Segal, M.R., Neuhaus, J.M., James, I.R. 1997: Dependence estimation for marginal models of multivariate survival data. *Lifetime Data Analysis* **3**, 251–268.

Senn, S. 1994: Testing for baseline balance in clinical trials. *Statistics in Medicine* **13**, 1715–1726.

Shah, B.V., Barwall, B.G. and Bieler, G.S. 1996: *SUDAAN user's manual, release 7.0*. Research Triangle Park, NC: Research Triangle Institute.

Shannon, H.S., and Szatmari, P. 1994: Seat-belt legislation and risk homeostasis: further analysis of the British data. *Accident Analysis & Prevention* **26**, 803–805.

Shao, J. 1990: Ordinary and weighted least-squares estimators. *Canadian Journal of Statistics* **18**, 327–336.

Shickle, D. and Chadwick, R. 1994: The ethics of screening: is 'screeningitis' an incurable disease? *Journal of Medical Ethics* **20**, 12–18.

Shipley, M.J., Smith, P.G. and Dramaix, M. 1989: Calculation of power for matched pair studies when randomization is by group. *International Journal of Epidemiology* **18**, 457–461.

Shirley, E.A.C. and Hickling, R. 1981: An evaluation of some statistical methods for analysing numbers of abnormalties found amongst litters in teratology studies. *Biometrics* **37**, 819–829.

Siddiqui, O., Hedeker, D., Flay, B. and Hu, F.B. 1996: Intraclass correlation in a school-based smoking prevention study – outcome and mediating variables, by sex and ethnicity. *American Journal of Epidemiology* **144**, 425–433.

Siddiqui, O., Mott, J., Anderson, T. and Flay, B. 1999: The application of Poisson random-effects regression models to the analyses of adolescents' current level of smoking. *Preventive Medicine* **29**, 91–101.

Silverman, W.A. and Chalmers, I. 1992: Sir Austin Bradford Hill: an appreciation. *Controlled Clinical Trials* **13**, 100–105.

Simon, R. 1981: Composite randomization designs for clinical trials. *Biometrics* **37**, 723–731.

Simon, R. 1982: Patient subsets and variation in therapeutic efficacy. *British Journal of Clinical Pharmacology* **14**, 473–482.

Simpson, J.M., Klar, N. and Donner, A. 1995: Accounting for cluster randomization: a review of primary prevention trials, 1990 through 1993. *American Journal of Public Health* **85**, 1378–1382.

Singer, J.D. 1998: Using SAS PROC MIXED to fit multilevel models, hierarchical models, and individual growth models. *Journal of Educational and Behavioral Statistics* **24**(4) 323–355.

Skrabanek, P. 1990: Why is preventive medicine exempted from ethical constraints? *Journal of Medical Ethics* **16**, 187–190.

Slymen, D.J. and Hovell, M.F. 1997: Cluster versus individual randomization in adolescent tobacco and alcohol studies: illustrations for design decisions. *International Journal of Epidemiology* **26**, 765–771.

Smith, P.J., Moffatt, M.E.K., Gelskey, S.C., Hudson, S. and Kaita, K. 1997: Are community health interventions evaluated appropriately? A review of six journals. *Journal of Clinical Epidemiology* **50**, 137–146.

Smith, P.J. and Morrow, R.H. 1991: *Methods for field trials of interventions against tropical diseases: a 'toolbox'*. Oxford: Oxford University Press.

Snedecor, G and Cochran, W. 1989: *Statistical methods*. 8th edn. Ames, Iowa: Iowa State University Press.

Sommer, A., Tarwotjo, I., Djunaedi, E., West, K.P. Jr, Loeden, A.A., Tilden, M.L. and the ACEH Study Group 1986: Impact of vitamin A supplementation on childhood mortality. *Lancet* **1**, May 24, 1169–1173.

Sorensen, G., Emmons, K., Hunt, M.K. and Johnson, D. 1998: Implications of the results of community intervention trials. *Annual Review of Public Health* **19**, 379–416.

Sorensen, G., Himmelstein, J.S., Hunt, M.K. *et al.* 1995: A model for worksite cancer prevention: integration of health protection and health promotion in the WellWorks project. *American Journal of Health Promotion* **10**, 55–62.

Sorensen, G., Thompson, B., Glanz, K. *et al.* 1996: Work site-based cancer prevention: primary results from the Working Well Trial. *American Journal of Public Health* **86**, 939–947.

Speed, T.P. 1991: Introduction to Fisher 1926: the arrangement of field experiments. In Kotz, S. and Johnson, N.L. (eds), *Breakthroughs in statistics*, vol. I. New York: Springer-Verlag.

Stanish, W.M. and Taylor, N. 1983: Estimation of the intraclass correlation coefficient for the analysis of covariance model. *American Statistician* **37**, 221–224.

Stansfield, S.K., Muller, P.L., Leribours, G. and Augustin, A. 1993: Vitamin A supplementation and increased prevalence of childhood diarrhea and acute respiratory infections. *Lancet* **342**, 578–582.

Stanton, B.F., Clemens, J.D. 1987: An educational intervention for altering water-sanitation behaviors to reduce childhood diarrhea in urban Bangladesh. *American Journal of Epidemiology* **125**, 292–301.

StataCorp. 1997: *Stata reference manual, Stata statistical software: release 5.0*. College Station, Texas: Stata Corporation.

Stewart-Brown, S. and Farmer, A. 1997: Screening could seriously damage your health. *British Medical Journal* **314**, 533–534.

Stigler, S.M. 1980: Stigler's law of eponymy. *Transactions of the New York Academy of Science* **30**, 147–157.

Stigler, S.M. 1986: *The history of statistics: the measurement of uncertainty before 1900*. Cambridge, MA: Belknap Press of Harvard University Press.

Strasser, T., Jeanneret, O. and Raymond, L. 1987: Ethical aspects of prevention trials, In Doxiadis, S. (ed.), *Ethical dilemmas in health promotion*. New York: John Wiley, Ch. 15.

Susser, M. 1985: Epidemiology in the United States after World War II: the evolution of technique. *Epidemiologic Reviews* **7**, 147–177.

Susser, M. 1995: Editorial: The tribulations of trials – intervention in communities. *American Journal of Public Health* **85**, 156–158.

Tang, D-I, Geller, N.L. and Pocock, S.J. 1993: On the design and analysis of randomized clinical trials with multiple endpoints. *Biometrics* **49**, 23–30.

Ten Have, T.R., Landis, J.R. and Hartzel, J. 1996: Population-averaged and cluster-specific models for clustered ordinal response data. *Statistics in Medicine* **15**, 2573–2588.

Thompson, B., Leynseele, J. and Beresford, S.A.A. 1997a: Recruiting worksites to participate in a health promotion research study. *American Journal of Health Promotion* **11**, 344–351.

Thompson, S.G., Pyke, S.D.M. and Hardy, R.J. 1997b: The design and analysis of paired cluster randomized trials: an application of meta-analysis techniques. *Statistics in Medicine* **16**, 2063–2980.

Torgerson, D.J. and Roland, M. 1998: What is Zelen's design? *British Medical Journal* **316**, 606.

Tuomilehto, J., Nissinen, A., Salonen, J.T., Kottke, T.E. and Puska, P. 1980: Community programme for control of hypertension in North Karelia, Finland. *Lancet* **2**, 900–903.

Turpeinen, O., Karvonen, M.J., Pekkarinen, M., Miettinen, M., Elosuo, R. and Paavilainen, E. 1979: Dietary prevention of coronary heart disease: the Finnish mental hospital study. *International Journal of Epidemiology* **8**, 99–118.

Ukoumunne, O.C., Gulliford, M.C., Chinn, S., Sterne, J.A.C., and Donner, A. 1998: Evaluation of health care interventions at area and organization level. In Black, N.A., Brazier, J., Fitzpatrick, R. and Reeves, B. (eds), *Health services research methods: a guide to best practice*. London: BMJ Books, 117–128.

Vachon, C.M., Sellers, T.A., Kushi, L.H. and Folsom, A.R. 1998: Familial correlation of dietary intakes among postmenopausal women. *Genetic Epidemiology* **15**, 553–563.

Vaeth, M. 1979: A note on the behaviour of occurrence/exposure rates when the survival distribution is not exponential. *Scandanavian Journal of Statistics* **6**, 77–80.

van Poppel, M.N.M., Koess, B.W., van der Ploeg, T., Smid, T. and Bouter, L.M. 1998: Lumbar supports and education for the prevention of low back pain in industry. A randomized trial. *Journal of the American Medical Association* **279**, 1789–1794.

Vartianinen, E., Puska, P., Jousilahti, P., Korhonen, H.J., Tuomilehto, J. and Nissinen, A. 1995: Twenty-year trends in coronary risk factors in North Karelia and in other areas of Finland. *International Journal of Epidemiology* **23**, 495–504.

Verbeke, G. 1997: Linear mixed models for longitudinal data. In Verbeke, G. and Molenberghs, G. (eds), *Linear mixed models in practice. A SAS-oriented approach.* New York: Springer-Verlag, Ch. 3.

Verma, V. and Le, T. 1996: An analysis of sampling errors for the demographic and health surveys. *International Statistical Review* **64**, 265–294.

Villar, J., Bakketeig, L., Donner, A. *et al.* 1998: The WHO antenatal care randomised trial: rationale and study design. *Paediatric and Perinatal Epidemiology* **12** (Suppl. 2), 27–58.

Villar, J. and Bergsjo, P. 1997: Scientific basis for the content of routine antenatal care. *Acta Obstetricia et Gynecologica Scandinavica* **76**, 1–14.

von Korff, M., Koepsell, T., Curry, S. and Dieher, P. 1992: Multi-level analysis in epidemiologic research on health behaviors and outcomes. *American Journal of Epidemiology* **135**, 1077–1082.

Voorhees, C.C., Stillman, F.A., Swank, R.T., Heagerty, P.J., Levine, D.M. and Becker, D.M. 1996: Heart, body, and soul: impact of church-based smoking cessation interventions on readiness to quit. *Preventive Medicine* **25**, 277–285.

Waller, L.A. 1997: A note on Harold S. Diehl, randomization, and clinical trials. *Controlled Clinical Trials* **18**, 180–183.

Walker, R., Heller, R., Redman, S., O'Connell, D. and Boulton, J. 1992: Reduction of ischemic heart disease risk markers in the teenage children of heart attack patients. *Preventive Medicine* **21**, 616–629.

Walsh, J.E. 1947: Concerning the effect of intraclass correlation on certain significance tests. *Annals of Mathematical Statistics* **18**, 88–96.

Walsh, M.W., Hilton, J.F., Masouredis, C.M., Gee, L., Chesney, M.A. and Ernster, V.L. 1999: Spit tobacco cessation intervention for college athletes: results after one year. *American Journal of Public Health* **89**, 228–234.

Ware, J.H. and Liang, K.Y. 1996: The design and analysis of longitudinal studies: a historical perspective. In Armitage, P. and David, H.A. (eds), *Advances in biometry*. New York: John Wiley, 339–362.

Wei, L.J., Su, J.Q. and Lachin, J.M. 1990: Interim analyses with repeated measurements in a sequential clinical trial. *Biometrika* **77**, 359–364.

Weil, C.S. 1970: Selection of the valid number of sampling units and a consideration of their combination in toxicological studies involving reproduction, teratogenesis or carcinogenesis. *Food and Cosmetics Toxicology* **8**, 177–182.

West, K.P., Pokhrel, R.P., Katz, J. *et al.* 1991: Efficacy of vitamin A in reducing preschool child mortality in Nepal. *Lancet* **338**, 67–71.

White, P.T., Pharoach, C.A., Anderson, H.R. and Freeling, P. 1987: Improving the outcome of chronic asthma in general practice: a randomized controlled trial of small group education. *Journal of the Royal College of General Practitioners* **39**, 182–186.

Whiting-O'Keefe, Q.E., Henke, C. and Simborg, D.W. 1984: Choosing the correct unit of analysis in medical care experiments. *Medical Care* **22**, 1101–1114.

Wilde, G.J.S. 1994: *Target risk: dealing with the danger of death, disease and damage in everyday decisions.* Toronto: PDE Publications.

Williams, D.A. 1975: The analyses of binary responses from toxicological experiments involving reproduction and teratogenicity. *Biometrics* **31**, 949–952.

Williams, D.A. 1982: Extra-binomial variation in logistic linear models. *Applied Statistics* **31**, 144–148.

Williams, D.H. and Davis, C.E. 1994: Reporting of assignment methods in clinical trials. *Controlled Clinical Trials* **15**, 294–298.

Williams, R.L. 1995: Product-limit survival functions with correlated survival times. *Lifetime Data Analysis* **1**, 171–186.

Woolf, B. 1955: On estimating the relation between blood group and disease. *Annals of Human Genetics* **11**, 251–253

Woolson, R.F., Bean, J.A. and Rojas, P.B. 1986: Sample size for case-control studies using Cochran's statistic. *Biometrics* **42**, 927–932.

Worden, J.K., Solomon, L.J., Flynn, B.S. *et al.* 1990: A community-wide program in breast self-examination training and maintenance. *Preventive Medicine* **19**, 254–269.

World Health Organization European Collaborative Group. 1986: European collaborative trial of multifactorial prevention of coronary heart disease: final report on the 6-year results. *Lancet* **1**, 868–872.

World Health Organization Maternal Health and Safe Motherhood Programme 1994: World Health Organization partograph in management of labour. *Lancet* **343**, 1399–1404.

World Medical Association. 1997: World Medical Association Declaration of Helsinki, 1996. *Journal of the American Medical Association* **277**, 925–926.

Yang, M., Woodhouse, G. and Healy, M. 1998: *A user's guide to MlwiN, Multilevel Models Project*. London, UK: Institute of Education, University of London.

Ying, Z. and Wei, L.J. 1994: The Kaplan–Meier estimate for dependent failure time observations. *Journal of Multivariate Analysis* **50**, 17–29.

Yusuf, S., Held, P., Teo, K.K. and Toretsky, E.R. 1990: Selection of patients for randomized controlled trials: implications of wide or narrow eligibility criteria. *Statistics in Medicine* **9**, 73–86.

Zapka, J.G., Costanza, M.E., Harris, D.R. *et al.* 1993: Impact of a breast cancer screening community intervention. *Preventive Medicine* **22**, 34–53.

Zelen, M. 1979: A new design for randomized clinical trials. *New England Journal of Medicine* **300**, 1242–1245.

Zelen, M. 1982: Strategy and alternate randomized designs in cancer clinical trials. *Cancer Treatment Reports* **66**, 1095–1100.

Zelen M. 1990: Randomized consent designs for clinical trials: an update. *Statistics in Medicine* **9**, 645–656.

Zhou, X.H., Perkins, A.J. and Hui, S.L. 1999: Comparisons of software packages for generalized linear multilevel models. *American Statistician* **53**, 282–290.

Ziegler, A., and Gromping, U. 1998: The generalised estimating equations: a comparison of procedures available in commercial statistical software packages. *Biometrical Journal* **40**, 245–260.

Zucker, D.M. 1990: An analysis of variance pitfall: the fixed effects analysis in a nested design. *Educational and Psychological Measurement* **50**, 731–738.

Zucker, D.M., Lakatos, E., Webber, L.S. *et al.* for the CATCH Study Group, 1995: Statistical design of the child and adolescent trial for cardiovascular health (CATCH): Implications of cluster randomization. *Controlled Clinical Trials* **16**, 96–118.

# Index